Handbook of Wet Age-Related Macular Degeneration

Tarek S. Hassan
George A. Williams

 Wolters Kluwer | Lippincott Williams & Wilkins
Health

Philadelphia • Baltimore • New York • London
Buenos Aires • Hong Kong • Sydney • Tokyo

Acquisitions Editor: Johathan Pine
Project Manager: Jennifer Jett
Manufacturing Manager: Jennifer Jett
Production Services: Maryland Composition
Printer: Walsworth Publishing Company

Figures 25–50 courtesy of Genentech.

530 Walnut Street
Philadelphia, Pennsylvania 19106 USA

351 West Camden Street
Baltimore, Maryland 21201-2436 USA

The publisher is not responsible (as a matter of product liability, negligence or otherwise) for an injury resulting from any material contained herein. This publication contains information relating to general principles of medical care which should not be constructed as specific instruction for individual patients. Manufacturer's product information should be reviewed for current information, including contraindications, dosages, and precautions.

Printed in the United States of America

Library of Congress Cataloging-in-Publication Data

Handbook of wet AMD / editors, Tarek S. Hassan, George A. Williams.
    p. ; cm.
ISBN-13: 978-0-7817-7148-1
1. Retinal degeneration—Age factors. I. Hassan, Tarek S. II. Williams, George A. (George Arthur), 1952- III. Title: Handbook of wet age-related macular degeneration.
[DNLM: 1. Macular Degeneration. WW 270 H236 2007]
RE661.D3H37 2007
617.7'35—dc22
            2007018973

The publishers have made every effort to trace copyright holders for borrowed material. If they have inadvertently overlooked any, they will be pleased to make the necessary arrangements at the first opportunity.

To purchase additional copies of this book, call our customer service department at (800) 638-3030 or fax orders to (301) 223-2320. For other book services, including chapter reprints and large quantity sales, ask for the Special Sales department.

For all other calls originating outside of the United States, please call (301) 223-2300.

Visit Lippincott Williams & Wilkins on the Internet: http://www.lww.com. Lippincott Williams & Wilkins customer service representatives are available from 8:30 am to 6:30 pm, EST, Monday through Friday, for telephone access.

10 9 8 7 6 5 4 3 2 1

TABLE OF CONTENTS

FOREWORD

Tarek S. Hassan

In the past several years, patients suffering from wet age-related macular degeneration (AMD) have been given new hope that their potential vision loss from this debilitating disease may be stemmed, and even somewhat reversed, in a striking reversal of fortune in the management of retinal disease. Only a few short years ago, a patient diagnosed with this potentially blinding disease could anticipate nearly certain vision loss as the best available treatments were only able to slow the progress of the disease–not reverse its impact on visual function. An explosion of interest and discovery has recently ushered in breakthroughs in early and improved diagnostic techniques and more successful treatment regimens that have fundamentally changed the retinal community's approach to this disease. Treating physicians and patients alike now share goals for outcomes never seen before: to reasonably expect *stabilization* of vision and to appropriately hope for *improvement* of vision following treatment for wet AMD.

Wet macular degeneration is being attacked on all fronts. From gaining a greater determination of incidences and prevalence to understanding more about risk factors, researchers and practitioners are developing an enhanced sense of the epidemiology of the disease. Knowing "where we've been" in treating the disease lays the groundwork for the development of future treatment directions. From a broader and more in-depth evaluation of the economic costs of the disease and its treatment comes the ability to more appropriately view the socioeconomic impact of research and development of therapeutic agents and techniques and their distribution to, and usage by, the many afflicted patients in our public health system, and the reimbursement for such intervention. From the breakthroughs achieved in elucidating details of the biochemistry of the development of wet AMD and the genetics of the disease in general, come the dramatic new treatments such as the use of intravitreal anti-vascular endothelial growth factor (VEGF) agents that have reversed the tide in the battle against vision loss, and the hopeful promise that new treatments are in sight that will lead to a cure for the affected and prevention for those at risk.

Introduction

Tarek S. Hassan

Age-related macular degeneration (AMD) is the leading cause of severe irreversible vision loss in developed nations and the third leading overall cause of blindness in the world (1,2). Currently, *advanced* AMD affects 25 to 30 million people worldwide and 1.75 million in the United States. The prevalence of advanced AMD is expected to rise, likely to affect roughly 3 million people in the United States by 2020 (3). At present, approximately 8 million Americans have at least *intermediate* AMD, and are thus at significant risk for progressing to more advanced vision loss during their lifetime (3).

The prevalence of AMD is affected by a number of factors, though none as significantly as advancing age. It is seen in some form in 8.5% of those 43 to 54 years old, approximately 30% of those 75 years and older, and nearly 50% of those 85 years and older (4,5). As life expectancy among people living in industrialized nations continues to increase, AMD will assuredly become an even greater public health problem in the future. The average life expectancy of an American born in 1900 was 47 years, while at present that same American would be expected to live approximately 78 years. In 2000, there were 35 million Americans aged 65 years and older, representing 12% of the U.S. population. By 2050, there are expected to be over 80 million Americans aged 65 years and older, which will represent over 20% of the population at that time. Of this aging population, by percentage, those 85 years and older are expected to be the fastest growing group in the next half century as both preventative and therapeutic medicine improves at breakneck speed (6).

There are gender and racial differences in the prevalence of AMD. Women have a higher risk of neovascular (wet) AMD, particularly at older ages. In the Beaver Dam Eye Study, women 75 years and older had a higher incidence of neovascular AMD than men of the same age (7). Caucasians had a much higher prevalence of AMD than African Americans at all ages. Caucasians 80 years and older had a significant increase in the occurrence of AMD compared with younger Caucasians, but this higher prevalence among the elderly was not seen in African Americans where the prevalence was 2 or less percent across all age groups. This is compared with at least a 10 times higher prevalence in white Americans ≥85 years old (3) (Fig. 1).

The Beaver Dam Eye Study showed that over a 10-year period, the cumulative incidence of early AMD was 12.1%, late AMD was 2%, and progression of AMD along a 6-step scale was 11.2%. The 10-year incidence of visual impairment of those diagnosed with early AMD was 22%, twice that of those not diagnosed with AMD (5,7–9).

AMD can be devastating to visual acuity, reduce or eliminate functional independence, and ultimately take a tragic toll on both patient and society. Retinal specialists have sought effective treatments for this significantly debilitating disease for many years. Until the advent of new therapies in the past few years, neovascular AMD would be expected to lead to legal blindness in 70% of untreated eyes within 2 years of onset (10,11). Moreover, 42% of patients with one eye affected with neovascular AMD will be expected to develop the same condition in the other eye within 5 years. This prospective vision loss

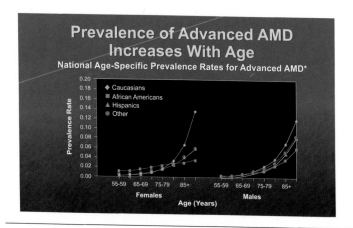

Figure 1. Comparative prevalence of advanced AMD: By increasing age and race. From Friedman DS, et al. *Vision problems in the US: Prevalence of adult vision impairment and age-related eye disease in America.* 4th ed. Prevent Blindness America; 2002. Available at http://www.preventblindness. org/vpus/VPUS_report_web.pdf. Accessed November 1, 2005, with permission.

is a significant personal and public health calamity toward which many resources have been applied, driven by the hope that successful treatments and, ultimately, a cure will be found. The past decade, and particularly the past few years, have seen dramatic breakthroughs in the pharmacologic management of AMD that have fundamentally changed the face of medical care for this disease. Patient and physician expectations for good outcomes have been vastly elevated, and the future looks even more promising.

The following sections will review many aspects of AMD including its characteristics; pathophysiology; past, current, and future treatment modalities; and socioeconomic impact as we present an overview of this potentially blinding disease.

Definition of AMD

AMD is a complex progressive disease characterized by macular cell damage, subsequent atrophy or exudation, and late-onset scarring. It is highly prevalent and may result in significant vision loss and functional disability of affected patients. Its clinical hallmark is the presence of *drusen*—yellowish sub-retinal deposits of metabolic waste products—and diffuse thickening of the basement membrane of the retinal pigment epithelium (RPE) and Bruch's membrane (Fig. 2). It is ultimately the premature dysfunction of the RPE that is the underlying defect in AMD. Two main types of AMD exist–the non-neovascular (dry) form that accounts for 90% of AMD cases, and the neovascular (wet) form that accounts for 10% of AMD cases but is responsible for 90% of the vision loss caused by the disease. Non-neovascular AMD, characterized by drusen, RPE rarefaction, and ultimately retinal atrophy, may remain static or be slowly progressive. Variable amounts of vision loss are seen depending on the location of

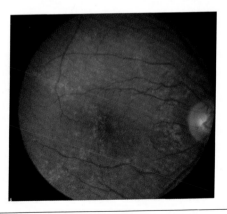

Figure 2. Extensive drusen in an eye with characteristic findings of AMD.

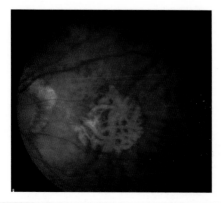

Figure 3. Non-neovascular AMD: Widespread geographic atrophy of the RPE.

the atrophic changes, worse with greater involvement of the foveal avascular zone (Fig. 3). Neovascular AMD is characterized by the development of choroidal neovascularization (CNV)–abnormal blood vessels that grow into the subretinal space from the choriocapillaris through defects in Bruch's membrane. These vessels are fragile and ultimately leak blood, fluid, and lipid into the subretinal space leading to symptoms of early vision loss (Fig. 4). The progressive growth of the neovascular network leads to disruption of Bruch's membrane, photoreceptors, and inner retina, and later to scarring and subsequent long-term permanent, vision loss. The resultant visual disability restricts or even prevents patients from being able to perform activities of daily living that include reading, driving, exercise, cooking, shopping, etc. Functional independence is impaired or lost, and this is often accompanied by great psychological distress. The collective diligence of researchers, practitioners, and pharmaceutical manufacturers, and the willingness of patients to participate in clinical trials have allowed for the development of new therapeutic options that have

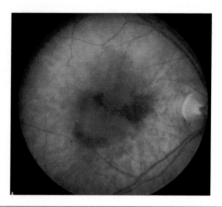

Figure 4. Neovascular AMD: Choroidal neovascularization with subretinal blood and fluid.

changed the focus of AMD treatment from the reduction of vision loss to visual improvement. Advances in our understanding of the epidemiology, natural history, pathophysiology, diagnostic measures, and ultimately treatments of AMD have led to advances that have been nothing short of monumental in our abilities to positively affect the lives of AMD patients.

Pathogenesis

George A. Williams

Although the pathogenesis of age-related macular degeneration (AMD) is enigmatic, recent information on the epidemiology and genetics of AMD provides valuable insight into the complex, multifactorial processes responsible for the development of AMD. It now seems likely that in most patients, AMD is the result of an interaction between genetic susceptibility and environmental risk factors (12). The elucidation of the details of this interaction is still preliminary but is beginning to explain the anatomic, epidemiologic, and clinical features that characterize AMD.

Pathology

Pathologic studies demonstrate that AMD is a disease of the choriocapillaris, Bruch's membrane, and retinal pigment epithelium (RPE) (13). The earliest clinical sign of AMD is the development of drusen. Drusen formation precedes both the geographic atrophy of the retinal pigment epithelium and the choroidal neovascularization (CNV) that characterize dry and wet AMD, respectively. Drusen consist of extracellular lipoproteinaceous deposits that accumulate between the RPE and Bruch's membrane (14–16). Concurrent with drusen formation, there is thickening and alteration of the filtration properties of Bruch's membrane (17). These changes compromise the ability of RPE to process photoreceptor disc membranes resulting in the formation of lipofuscin, a byproduct of incomplete outer segment processing. Lipofuscin accumulation in the RPE destabilizes cellular membranes, sensitizes the RPE to oxidative damage, and induces apoptosis resulting in RPE dysfunction or death (18).

The clinical appearance of drusen is dynamic. Drusen commonly change in size, shape, and location over months and years, perhaps reflecting the underlying metabolic turmoil in AMD. Although drusen have long been recognized as a risk factor for the development of CNV, it is unknown whether they contribute to the formation of CNV or represent an epiphenomenon. Recently, studies demonstrating the presence of complement components in human drusen and experimental CNV models suggest drusen promote CNV (19). Furthermore, the Beaver Dam Eye Study demonstrated that eyes with multiple small drusen (58) have an increased 15-year incidence of soft drusen, pigmentary abnormalities, and late AMD (26). However, in clinical trials, photocoagulation has been shown to decrease the number and size of drusen, but this does not decrease the formation of CNV (20,21). Therefore, the role of drusen in the formation of CNV remains to be definitively established.

The anatomic features of neovascular age-related macular degeneration are manifested by new blood vessel growth from the choroid through Bruch's membrane into the subretinal space. Three basic growth patterns of choroidal neovascularization have been described based upon the relationship of the CNV to the RPE. In type 1, the CNV is beneath the RPE. In type 2, the CNV is through the RPE and into the subretinal space. The combined pattern has both type 1 and type 2 CNV. There is some correlation between these growth patterns and clinical and fluorescein angiographic features. Type 1

CNV tends to have the clinical and angiographic features of occult CNV with a fibrovascular retinal pigment epithelium detachment. Type 2 CNV often has the clinical and angiographic features of classic CNV (15).

Another form of neovascular age-related macular degeneration is retinal angiomatous proliferation (RAP), which is characterized by early intraretinal neovascularization which may precede or occur simultaneously with choroidal neovascularization. This intraretinal neovascularization has distinct clinical and angiographic features including intraretinal hemorrhage and a focal area of hyperfluorescence on indocyanine green angiography. Typically the intraretinal neovascularization of RAP anastomoses with both retinal vessels and type 2 CNV (22).

Serous detachment of the retinal pigment epithelium (PED) is another feature of neovascular AMD. Serous PED is manifested clinically by a well-demarcated elevation of the retinal pigment epithelium, which anatomically corresponds to the accumulation of fluid between the RPE and Bruch's membrane. It is thought that this is due to the obstruction of the normal flow of fluid through the retina and RPE into the choroid by lipid deposits in Bruch's membrane. This lipid deposition decreases the passage of water through Bruch's membrane and forces fluid to accumulate beneath the RPE (23).

The end-stage of neovascular age-related macular degeneration is characterized by subretinal fibrosis, retinal detachment, and photoreceptor atrophy. This stage is commonly preceded by subretinal or subretinal pigment epithelium hemorrhage and is described clinically as a disciform scar.

Risk Factors

Epidemiologic studies have identified multiple risk factors for the development of AMD. The primary risk factor is, of course, age. The Eye Disease Prevalence Research Group estimated that advanced

AMD, defined as either geographic atrophy or neovascular AMD, is present in .05% of people 40 to 49 years of age and 11.8% of people 80 years of age or greater (24). The Beaver Dam Eye Study found an 8% prevalence rate for early AMD in people 43 to 54 years of age, which increased to 30% in people 75 years of age or greater (25). For late AMD, the prevalence was 0% in the younger group increasing to 7% in the older group. This study also demonstrated the development of AMD over time with 14% and 3% of people who did not have AMD at baseline developing early AMD and late AMD, respectively, over 15 years (26). The Blue Mountains Eye Study found a 10-year incidence of early and late AMD of 10.8% and 2%, respectively (27).

Race is also a risk factor for AMD. Studies indicate that AMD affects whites and Hispanics more commonly than blacks (24,28,29). The Eye Disease Prevalence Research Group demonstrated that among persons 80 years of age or greater, black men and women have the lowest prevalence of neovascular AMD, approximately 1% to 2%, compared with 8% to 11% for white men and women (30–32). The Age-Related Eye Diseases Study (AREDS) also found a lower incidence of neovascular AMD in blacks compared with whites (33). This may be related to the protective antioxidant effects of melanin on the RPE, Bruch's membrane, and photoreceptors. Although the incidence of neovascular AMD in blacks is lower, it is not negligible, and neovascular AMD must be considered as a cause for visual loss in blacks. The Beaver Dam Eye Study and the Blue Mountains Eye Study demonstrated women to be more likely to develop early and late AMD (25,34). However, other studies have not confirmed this association between gender and AMD prevalence (28,33,35). Regardless of whether gender is a risk factor for the development of AMD, there is no evidence that gender has any effect on the response to treatment.

Age, gender, and race constitute unchangeable risk factors. Multiple modifiable risk factors have also been correlated with AMD. These factors are important from a treatment perspective since appropriate intervention may affect disease progression. The following modifiable risk factors have been associated with the development and progression of AMD: cigarette smoking, blood pressure, pulse pressure, lipid levels, abdominal obesity, physical activity, dietary fat, and cataract surgery (33). There is new, strong evidence that AMD is a complex genetic disease in which there is important interaction between genetic and modifiable risks factors (12,36). These relationships are discussed later, but they confirm the need for risk modification strategies in the management of AMD.

Perhaps the strongest modifiable risk factor is cigarette smoking (37). The mechanisms implicating cigarette smoking in the pathogenesis of AMD include direct toxicity to the RPE, damage to luteal pigment, decreased choroidal perfusion, oxidative damage, and immune activation. Multiple studies have identified both the presence and amount of cigarette smoking to be correlated with the prevalence of early and advanced AMD (38,39). The Nurses' Health Study found a positive correlation between the prevalence of AMD and the number of cigarettes smoked (40). In the AREDS, individuals with more than 10 pack years of smoking had an increased risk of neovascular AMD and central GA with odds ratios of 1.5 and 1.79, respectively (33). However, in the Beaver Dam Eye Study, among patients who quit smoking between the baseline and 5-year follow-up, there was no decrease in the subsequent risk of AMD compared with those who continued to smoke (32). Although these epidemiologic data do not definitely prove that stopping smoking prevents the development of advanced AMD, this is yet another reason that patients should be advised not to smoke.

Several studies have demonstrated blood pressure to be a risk factor for AMD (30,41,42). This may be related to the adverse effects of hypertension on the choroidal vasculature. In the Beaver Dam Eye Study, persons with treated and controlled hypertension at baseline and those with uncontrolled hypertension at baseline were approximately two and three times as likely, respectively, to develop neovascular AMD over the 10-year follow-up as normotensive persons (43).

Also, an increase of greater than 5 mm Hg in systolic blood pressure over the first 5 years of the study increased the risk of developing late AMD by 3.5 fold. Although other studies including the AREDS have not confirmed that hypertension is a risk factor for AMD, appropriate blood pressure control is prudent (33,42,44,45).

Dyslipidemia is an inconsistent risk factor for AMD. Some studies report a correlation with serum high density lipoprotein while others do not (33,44,45). The use of statins to modify lipid profiles has been correlated with a lower risk of AMD in some studies but not others (46–48). Putative mechanisms for a possible beneficial effect of statins include diminished accumulation of lipids in Bruch's membrane, antioxidant effects, and inhibition of endothelial apoptosis. However, larger studies have failed to confirm a beneficial effect for AMD by statins (42,49).

Greater body mass has been associated with a higher risk of AMD progression. One study demonstrated an association between greater waist-hip ratio and waist circumference as measures of abdominal adiposity and basal metabolic index (50). The AREDS found greater body mass to be associated with GA (33). Obesity may be a marker for reduced physical activity, which has been correlated with neovascular AMD. However, other studies have not confirmed this association, and one study correlated lean body mass with an increased risk of GA.

There is increasing evidence that diet is an important modifiable risk factor for AMD (51–53). Higher total fat intake increases the risk of progression to advanced AMD. Both animal and vegetable saturated, monounsaturated, polyunsaturated, and transunsaturated fats increase the risk of progression (52). Conversely, diets high in omega 3 fatty acids from fish appears to lower the risk of AMD progression (52,54,55). The potential benefits of omega 3 fatty acids are being evaluated in a randomized clinical trial, AREDS II (areds2.org).

The association between cataract surgery and progression of AMD is a controversial but important question because of the common association of both early AMD and cataract in elderly persons (56,57). In the Beaver Dam Eye Study, 27% of persons older than 75 years of age had both cataract and early AMD in at least one eye at baseline (58). A pooled analysis from two large population-based studies, the Beaver Dam and the Blue Mountains, demonstrated a 5.7 times higher risk for the development of either GA or CNV in nonphakic eyes compared with phakic eyes (59). A recent retrospective observational population-based case-control study used photodynamic therapy as a marker for neovascular AMD in patients also undergoing cataract surgery. The study demonstrated an increase in the frequency of PDT in the first 6 months after cataract surgery and between 12 and 18 months after cataract surgery compared with controls (59). These studies support the hypothesis that cataract surgery increases the risk of developing neovascular AMD. However, in the prospective AREDS there was a nonsignificant association between cataract surgery and progression to advanced AMD (59b). Regardless of the role of cataract surgery in the progression of AMD, most patients with AMD and visually significant cataract note an improvement in quality of life independent of AMD severity (60). It is important for ophthalmologists to discuss with patients the controversial association of AMD progression and cataract surgery (61,62).

The Role of Genetics in AMD

A genetic predisposition for the development of AMD has long been recognized, and the presence of a positive family history for AMD is a strong risk factor for AMD. Familial aggregation studies, twin studies, and segregation analysis provide strong evidence for a genetic component in AMD (63,64). In a study of first-degree relatives (mostly siblings) of 119 AMD cases, the prevalence of AMD was significantly higher among the relatives of the AMD cases than among the relatives of controls, (23.7% vs. 11.6%) with an age and sex adjusted odds ratio of 2.4 (95% confidence interval [CI] 1.2 to 4.7).

Among relatives of the cases with neovascular AMD, the odds ratio (OR) was 3.1 (95% CI, 1.5–6.7) (65). Twin studies also suggest genetic factors play a substantial role in the etiology of AMD and may explain 46% to 71% of the variation in the severity of the disease (66). Advanced disease may have higher heritability.

In 2005, the simultaneous publication of three reports describing a genetic mutation in the complement factor H (CFH) gene on chromosome 1 heralded a breakthrough in the understanding of the pathogenesis of AMD (67–69). The first genetic defect identified was the single nucleotide polymorphism (SNP) Y402H. Subsequently, other variants in complement factor H gene have been reported (12). A second AMD associated mutation has been identified on chromosome 10q 26 (70,71). This is identified as LOC387715 and involves SNP A69S. The gene HTRA 1 has been implicated (12). The variants of CFH and LOC387715 appear to account for up to 63% of the population attributable risk for AMD.

A meta-analysis indicates that the risk allele for CFH has an OR of 2.4 (95% CI, 2.2–2.7) and 6.2 (95% CI, 5.4–7.2) in the heterozygous and homozygous states, respectively. For LOC387715, the OR for heterozygous and homozygous states are 2.5 (95% CI, 2.2–2.9) and 7.3 (95% CI, 5.7–9.4), respectively. The joint contribution of homozygous complement factor H Y402H and LOC387715 produce an odds ratio of 57.6 for development of AMD compared with controls. However, the presence of mutation does not guarantee the development of AMD nor does the absence eliminate all risks. The CFH Y402H allele and LOC387715 allele are present in 58% and 34% of the white U.S. population. In persons with advanced AMD, 18% do not have the CFH high-risk allele. Similarly, in persons without any evidence of AMD, there are one or two copies of the high-risk CFH allele in 45.4% and 10.7% of individuals, respectively. This confirms the complex genetic nature of AMD (12,36,71–73).

Importantly, it has been shown that these two gene variants interact with modifiable risk factors to further increase the risk of AMD.

Multiple studies show both smoking and obesity increase the risks associated with these variants (39,73). In one study, subjects homozygous for CFH Y402H had a 12-fold increase risk if they were obese and a 9-fold increase with smoking. For LOC387715 A69S homozygotes, the increased risks were 9-fold and 22-fold for obesity and smoking, respectively (73).

Such studies have raised questions concerning the potential value of population-based genetic screening (12,36,73,74). Positive screening may be useful in convincing some individuals to alter modifiable risk factors such as smoking and obesity or access more frequent eye screening. However, the high prevalence of these variants in the general populations implies a relative low positive predictive value for genetic testing. If more effective preventative strategies for AMD are developed, genetic testing may become more valuable.

The elucidation of the complement factor H polymorphism(s) and LOC387715 provides important insights into the pathogenesis of AMD (72,75). Complement factor H is an important regulatory protein in the alternative complement pathway that mediates inflammation. Dysfunctional complement factor H induces a pro-inflammatory state. The association of the complement component 2 and factor B genes in AMD further implicates the complement pathway. This strongly supports a major inflammatory component in the pathogenesis of AMD (76). The role of inflammation is supported by analysis of drusen demonstrating the presence of complement factors C5a, C3a, and CFH (19). Additionally, C reactive protein (CRP) and homocysteine have been associated with AMD (77–81). CRP and homocysteine are markers for both inflammation and atherosclerosis, lending further support to the role of inflammation in AMD. The combination of the complement factor H Y402H mutation and the inflammatory markers erythrocyte sedimentation rate and CRP increases the odds ratio for AMD to 20.2 and 27.7, respectively (81b). The HTRA1 gene encodes a serine protease that regulates degradation of the extracellular matrix proteoglycans. This proteolysis facilitates further breakdown of the extracellular matrix by collagenases and matrix metalloproteinases. This may result in destruction of Bruch's membrane, facilitating migration of neovascularization beneath the retinal pigment epithelium or retina (82). HTRA1 also inhibits transforming growth factor beta, which affects extracellular matrix formation and angiogenesis.

Thus, while the CFH Y402H polymorphism and LOC287715 variants account for over half of AMD, the risk of AMD is further increased in the presence of stimulation of the complement cascade, which may be related to environmental factors such as smoking, oxidation, and infection. This confirms the importance of altering modifiable risk factors whenever possible.

Pathobiology

Localized inflammation, perhaps in conjunction with ischemia affecting the choriocapillaris, RPE, and Bruch's membrane complex, may stimulate the production of vascular endothelial growth factor (VEGF), a potent vascular endothelial cell mitogen (13). VEGF is a homodimeric glycoprotein which was purified and cloned in 1989 (83,84). There are several VEGFs in the VEGF family of growth factors of which VEGF A is most relevant to AMD. Within VEGF A there are multiple isoforms identified by the number of amino acids constituting the protein. These include VEGF 206, VEGF 189, VEGF 165, VEGF 145, VEGF 121, and VEGF 120. The function of each isoform and the interplay between the isoforms is an area of active investigation. VEGF is expressed by most ocular tissues including the retina and RPE in response to ischemia and inflammation. VEGF is both sufficient and necessary for the development of both normal vasculogenesis and neovascularization (85,86). Also, and importantly for AMD, VEGF is a potent vascular permeability agent. Thus, VEGF is central to both the vessel growth and leakage that characterizes choroidal neovascularization. Both animal models and human tissue studies have established the importance of VEGF in the pathogenesis of CNV. VEGF is secreted by the basal RPE toward the choroid where high levels of the two VEGF receptors are located (85,86). The VEGF receptors 1 and 2 are tyrosine kinases which upon binding with VEGF initiate a cascade of molecular events resulting in angiogenesis and vascular personality. These events include breakdown of the extracellular matrix, endothelial cell replication and migration, and vessel formation. In addition, VEGF polymorphisms have been associated with neovascular AMD (87). Although VEGF is an integral factor in the pathogenesis of choroidal neovascularization, other growth factors and cytokines are also operative. Pigment epithelial derived factor (PEDF) is produced by the RPE and inhibits angiogenesis. PEDF and VEGF may act in concert to regulate angiogenesis. As choroidal neovascularization develops, matrix metalloproteins are produced to lyse the extracellular matrix, which allows the new vessels to migrate. The breakdown of the extracellular matrix releases plasminogen, fibrin, and platelet-derived growth factor, all of which contribute to angiogenesis. Thus, the active growth of choroidal neovascularization is characterized by a proteolytic state with endothelial cell duplication, migration, and organization into vascular channels. Hematopoietic stem cells may also be imported into the process. Eventually the active growth of choroidal neovascularization ceases and an involutional stage characterized by fibrosis begins. This fibrosis is correlated with the expression of antiproteolytic factors such as tissue inhibitors of matrix metalloproteinases and transforming growth factor beta. The clinical result is the formation of a disciform scar (15). The elucidation of the role of VEGF in CNV has revolutionized the treatment of neovascular AMD. Multiple potent anti-VEGF technologies, which will be discussed later, have been or are being developed.

Diagnosis

Tarek S. Hassan

The physical appearance of AMD has been described in many ways during the past 40 years. In its most basic consideration, AMD may be thought of as "dry" if it is non-neovascular or "wet" if it is associated with CNV. In recent years its characterization has evolved beyond this distinction and has become more relevant, however, as new treatments and preventative measures have been developed.

Presently, most classify AMD into 3 stages—*early, intermediate, or advanced*—based on clinically determined anatomic findings. Any stage may affect one or both eyes, and the more advanced stages evolve from earlier ones. This scheme was developed for use in the Age-Related Eye Disease Study (AREDS), which evaluated long-term clinical outcomes of eyes receiving nutritional supplements and placebo for prophylaxis against the progression of AMD. Extensive natural history data was also garnered from this trial. *Early AMD* is characterized the presence of extensive small drusen (<63 μm), or a few medium-sized drusen (63 μm–124 μm), and generally no significant visual symptoms (Fig. 5). Eyes with this stage are at low risk for developing significant visual loss with only a 1% chance of developing

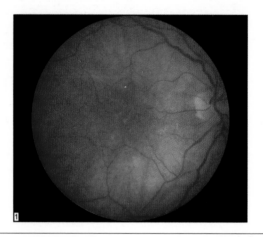

Figure 5. Early AMD with drusen.

advanced AMD. Eyes with *intermediate AMD* have numerous medium-sized drusen, at least one large druse (≥125 μm), or an area of geographic atrophy of the RPE that spares the center of the fovea (Fig. 6). Patients with this stage of AMD have either no visual complaints or mild vision loss, with or without metamorphopsia. They are at higher risk for progression to more severe vision loss; 18% develop advanced AMD within 5 years of diagnosis. *Advanced AMD* may be either non-neovascular or neovascular. Eyes with advanced non-neovascular AMD demonstrate geographic atrophy of the RPE, often involving the foveal center, as well as associated breakdown of the overlying photoreceptors that lead to significant vision loss in most affected patients (Fig. 7). Eyes with these manifestations in one eye have a 43% likelihood of progressing to advanced AMD in the fellow eye over the next 5 years.

Eyes with advanced neovascular AMD develop CNV through breaks in the damaged Bruch's membrane, and into the subretinal and sub-RPE spaces. These unstable vessels leak blood and fluid into

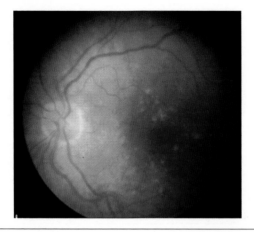

Figure 6. Intermediate AMD with numerous medium-sized drusen.

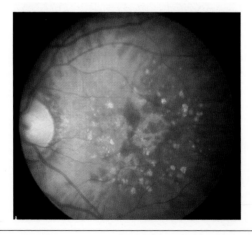

Figure 7. Advanced *Non-neovascular* AMD with large drusen and geographic RPE atrophy.

these regions that causes physical disruption to the retinal anatomy, including the photoreceptors, and to the visual conduction processes by the space-occupying nature of the lesions (Fig. 8). Significant central visual loss typically results (88).

CNV lesions have been characterized by both their location relative to the fovea and fluorescein angiographic characteristics. They may be extrafoveal, juxtafoveal, or subfoveal in location; subfoveal lesions are the most common. Angiographic classifications include predominantly classic, minimally classic, or occult, describing the pattern of fluorescein dye leakage. These features will be discussed further below in the section on diagnostic testing.

Diagnostic evaluation and workup

AMD is important to diagnose at any stage. When identified early, it allows for close follow-up by eye specialists to better detect progres-

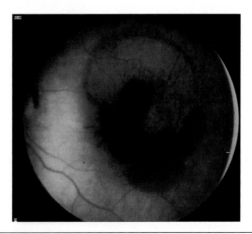

Figure 8. Advanced *Neovascular* AMD with subretinal hemorrhage and fluid.

sion at its earliest stages. When seen later in its course, AMD, particularly in the neovascular form, may be treated with recently approved medications that are successful at either stabilizing or improving vision to a degree not seen prior to the last couple of years. Specific nutritional supplementation given to patients with these findings may be prophylactic in reducing the likelihood of further vision loss in the fellow eye (88). As treatment and preventative techniques improve, it becomes increasingly important to diagnose and follow AMD even at its earliest stages.

Patient Evaluation

A dilated funduscopic examination is ultimately required to diagnose AMD, although the initial patient encounter, including a good medical history, may provide early clues to its presence. Patients note a range of visual symptoms depending on the severity of disease, from no visual complaints to mild to severe decreased vision, metamorphopsia, and scotomas. Patients may report difficulty reading, telling time, driving, watching television, recognizing faces, using the telephone, and the like. They may report abnormalities identified with the use of an Amsler grid on which new distortion or losses of areas of recognition are seen.

Visual function is generally assessed using either a standard Snellen acuity chart or an Early Treatment Diabetic Retinopathy Study (ETDRS) chart to determine distance visual acuity. Near visual acuity is more affected in many patients if AMD involves the foveal avascular zone, and thus it is a less sensitive and helpful measure of visual functioning. Most controlled clinical trials use standardized ETDRS acuity charts. Although obviously important in the assessment of the AMD patient, visual acuity alone may underestimate the disability caused by the disease particularly if the fovea is spared. The National Eye Institute's Visual Function Questionnaire (NEI-VFQ) has been shown to be an effective supplemental measure to better assess visual function. It reflects how quality of life indicators change over time with incremental changes in visual acuity. For example, a three-line visual acuity change equals a 7-point NEI-VFQ score change. A 5-point decrease in the overall NEI-VFQ score reflects a significant worsening of visual function (89). This method of tracking visual function is not used in standard clinical practice but offers insight into the ultimate effects of the disease on patient lifestyles. It can be used to better quantitate the socioeconomic outcomes of both the natural history of, and treatments for, AMD-induced visual decrease.

Changes in contrast sensitivity occur with progression of AMD. They correlate with the ability to perform mobility and recognition tasks and represent another useful measure of visual function, although tests of contrast sensitivity are not commonly performed in most office situations outside of controlled clinical trials. A six-letter loss of contrast sensitivity represents approximately the same level of functional decrease as a 15-letter loss of ETDRS vision (90,91). Reading speed, testable by several methods, similarly correlates with visual functioning (92). Significant visual acuity and functional loss from AMD is often caused by absolute or relative scotomas (Fig 9). These may not be assessed well by most measures of vision testing, but their size and location can be accurately demonstrated by macular perimetry with a scanning laser ophthalmoscope (SLO) (93–95).

Though generally thought of as a patient self-examination tool, an Amsler grid may be used by the clinician in lieu of more sophisticated SLO testing to identify scotomas. Patients are asked to describe, quantitate if possible, and note changes in, or absence of, the lines that surround the central dot (Fig. 10). The newly developed Preferential Hyperacuity Perimeter (PHP) is a more sophisticated electronic form of an Amsler grid that allows for more precise mapping of scotomas and potentially earlier detection of new-onset CNV (96). Clinical trials to evaluate the benefits of the PHP are ongoing.

When the patient comes to medical attention, clinical funduscopic examination using slit lamp biomicroscopy with a macular viewing lens is the gold standard for highly sensitive and specific detection of

Decreased Vision

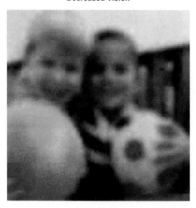

Central or Paracenteral Scotoma

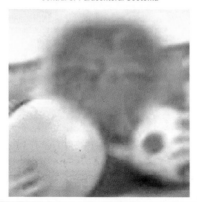

Figure 9. Representation of decreased vision and scotoma from advanced AMD. From National Eye Institute. National Institutes of Health. Available at http://www.nei.nih.gov/photo/sims/index.asp and http://www.nei.nih.gov/photo/charts/index.asp. Accessed November 1, 2005, with permission.

Distortion

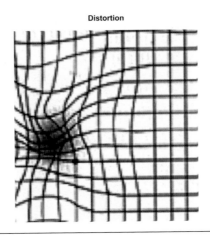

Figure 10. Amsler grid distortion seen by a patient with choroidal neovascularization. From National Eye Institute. National Institutes of Health. Available at http://www.nei.nih.gov/photo/sims/index.asp and http://www.nei.nih.gov/photo/charts/index.asp. Accessed November 1, 2005, with permission.

abnormalities. Drusen, RPE atrophy, with or without hyperpigmentation, subretinal blood and/or fluid, or some combination of these features is typically seen.

Once these features are identified clinically, ancillary studies are employed to determine if CNV is present, and then to characterize the size, type, and other features of the abnormal blood vessel complex if found. They also demonstrate the presence and amount of subretinal fluid, intraretinal fluid and/or cystoid macular edema, pigment epithelial detachment (PED), and RPE atrophy, allowing for effective monitoring of treatment responses. Current gold standard studies include fluorescein angiography (FA) and optical coherence tomography (OCT). Indocyanine green (ICG) angiography is also helpful in identifying lesions in the deeper choroid but is less often used in most

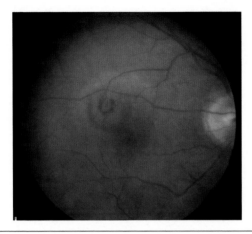

Figure 11. Extrafoveal choroidal neovascularization, color photograph.

clinical settings. Fluorescein does not penetrate healthy RPE or leak from normal retinal vasculature, and thus FA is successful at demonstrating the presence, location, size, and composition of CNV—all of which have implications relative to potential treatment strategies.

The location of the CNV is most important in assessing the impact the lesion has on vision and determining potential options for treatment. Choroidal neovascularization is classified as *extrafoveal* if it is ≥200 μm from the center of the foveal avascular zone (FAZ) (Fig. 11), *juxtafoveal* if ≥1 μm but <200 μm from the center of the FAZ (Fig. 12), and *subfoveal* when any aspect of the lesion involves the geometric center of the FAZ (Fig. 13) (97–99). Most patients who present for treatment of AMD-related vision loss have subfoveal lesions. Zawinka and coworkers reported that in an urban population, 76% of newly diagnosed CNV were subfoveal, 15% were juxtafoveal, and 6% were extrafoveal (100).

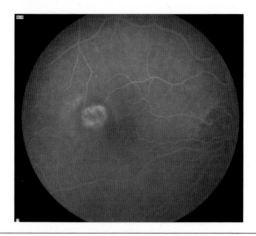

Figure 12. Juxtafoveal choroidal neovascularization, fluorescein angiography.

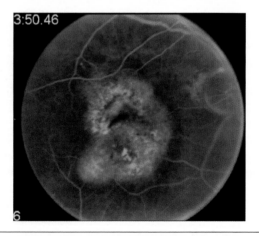

Figure 13. Subfoveal choroidal neovascularization, fluorescein angiography.

Lesion size and progression are important features to follow. In the Macular Photocoagulation Study (MPS), CNV was measured in units of disc areas (DA). More recently, clinicians use the greatest linear dimension (GLD)–defined as the greatest distance between two points on the boundary of the CNV divided by the magnification of the image from which the measurement is taken. For example, a lesion with a GLD measured to be 10 mm on a 35 mm film image magnified 2.5 times is considered to be 4 mm in actual size (101). Digital FA software packages are now able to calculate GLD directly from the original images. A treating physician needs an accurate assessment of lesion size to determine proper laser spot sizes when photodynamic therapy (PDT) is employed and to note the changes that occur with the natural history of the lesion or with response to therapy. Recent disease progression, illustrated as lesion growth, has been defined as new blood associated with CNV, growth of the GLD by ≥10% within the prior 3 months, and/or loss of 1 line of vision in the prior 3 months (101).

The composition of the CNV lesion can be determined by careful analysis of the entire sequence of the FA and the components of the neovascular process classified as either classic or occult.

FA characteristics (102)

Classic CNV

Early phase: Bright choroidal hyperfluorescence with well-demarcated borders; actual vessel visualization not required (Fig. 14A).

Later phases: Increasing accumulation of fluorescein in the subretinal space, beyond borders seen in the early phases, that obscures CNV margins (Fig. 14B).

Occult CNV

Two patterns that exist alone or in combination

Fibrovascular PED (FVPED):

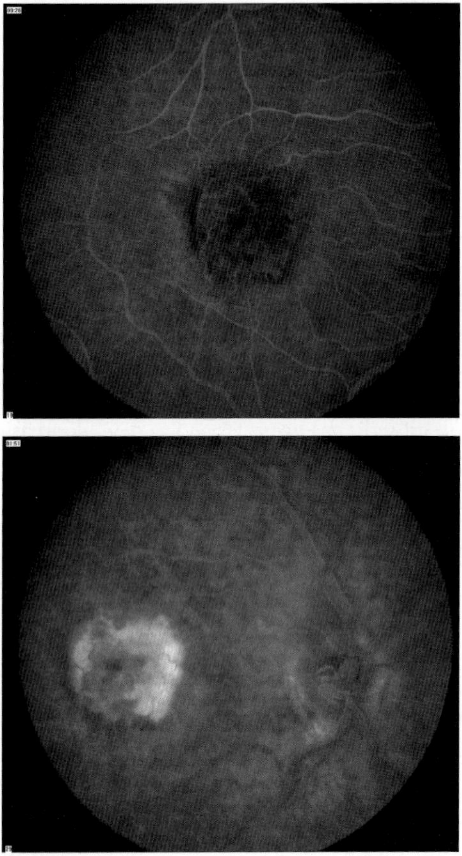

Figure 14. **A.** Classic subfoveal CNV: Early fluorescein angiographic image. **B.** Classic subfoveal CNV: Mid-late fluorescein angiographic image.

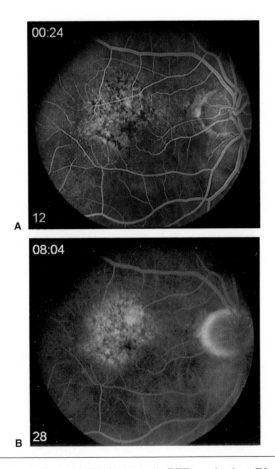

Figure 15. **A.** Occult CNV–fibrovascular PED: early phase FA.
B. Occult CNV–fibrovascular PED: late phase FA.

Early phase: Irregular RPE elevation with speckled, moderately bright hyperfluorescence appearing within 2 minutes of dye injection (Fig. 15A).

Later phases: By 10 minutes after injection, moderate, persistent, poorly demarcated hyperfluorescent staining or leakage into the subretinal space (Fig. 15B).

■ Note: Typical serous PEDs appear different by FA, seen as smooth elevations of the RPE with early, well-demarcated uniform hyperfluorescence that persists in the late phases.

Late leakage of an undetermined source (LLUS):

Early phase: No sign of either classic or FVPED; no source of leakage is evident (Fig. 16A).

Late phases: By 2 to 5 minutes post-injection, poorly demarcated and speckled dye leakage is seen that is not noted early (Fig. 16B).

■ Note: A well-demarcated area of hyperfluorescence is NOT synonymous with classic CNV nor is a poorly demarcated lesion synonymous with occult CNV.

Analysis of FA characteristics may be complicated by the presence of several features that may make it difficult to interpret the size, distribution, and type of lesion: thick blood, hyperplastic RPE or fibrous tissue, and serous PED. When evaluating the association of visible blood with the lesion, it is customary to determine if the blood is a "component" of, or "associated" with, the CNV. As a CNV *component*, it may obscure visualization of the CNV boundaries and its distribution is included as part of the total lesion size. Blood *associated* with the CNV is found in the sub-RPE, subretinal, intraretinal, or preretinal spaces, and does not obscure the borders of the lesion (103). A determination of whether hyperplastic RPE and/or fibrous tissue is part

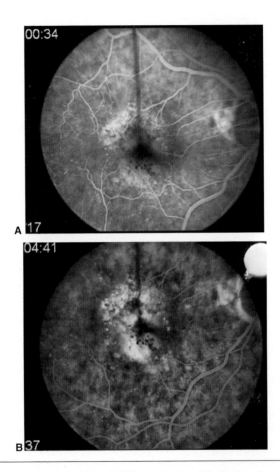

Figure 16. **A.** Occult CNV–LLUS: early phase FA. **B.** Occult
CNV–LLUS: late phase FA.

of the lesion or not is similarly important when considering total CNV size and activity. A serous PED is felt to be a lesion component if it is seen adjacent to CNV elements. Its own hyperfluorescence may obscure that of the underlying CNV, and thus its dimensions are considered part of the total lesion (104).

After identifying and assessing all lesion components, the treating physician may then classify the CNV based on its composition as either classic, minimally classic, or occult (101):

Predominantly classic CNV: Classic CNV component makes up ≥50% of the entire lesion (Fig. 14).

Minimally classic CNV: Classic component makes up 1%–49% of the entire lesion (Fig. 13).

Occult CNV: No classic component is seen (Fig. 15).

Though occult CNV is typically less aggressive than classic CNV, eyes with either occult or minimally classic lesions should be carefully monitored for progression to a predominantly classic subtype (105). The TAP (Treatment of Age-Related Macular Degeneration With Photodynamic Therapy) trial found a 40% rate of conversion of lesions classified as minimally classic at baseline to predominantly classic when they received no treatment, 21% doing so within 3 months (103). Fluorescein angiography provides vital information for the treating physician to clarify the nature of a specific CNV lesion and to aid in the application of clinical trial data to the decision-making process involved in choosing the appropriate therapeutic option among the increasing number of potential treatments. The interpretation of FA data is becoming more sophisticated, as are the techniques and instruments involved in performing the test and capturing the images. Special filters that highlight the unique spectral characteristics of photodynamic dyes may enhance FA visualization. Automated analytic image interpretation is being developed where images are pixilated and biocomputation methods are employed to evaluate areas of interest. Other automated image analysis methods are being developed that may soon be more specific and sensitive in characterizing disease and lesion components than human interpretation methods. Richard Rosen, MD, and coworkers have developed a custom device that can simultaneously superimpose three types of imaging to improve assessment of occult CNV and further expand our understanding of lesion characteristics. This second generation unit combines SLO, OCT, and ICG angiography to create an integrated image that provides an enhanced view of morphology and angiographic features that may lead to improved treatment of occult CNV. ICG angiography, though less commonly employed than FA, can give a view of the choroidal vessels rather than the retinal vasculature that is seen with FA. ICG is more completely bound to plasma proteins and fluoresces in the near-infrared portion of the light spectrum. This may be helpful when evaluating cases of pure occult CNV or if blood or highly elevated PED fluid obscures the view of the lesion architecture. It may also be useful when evaluating eyes with chorioretinal anastomosis, retinal angiomatous proliferation (RAP), or polypoidal choroidal vasculopathy (PCV) (106,107). In RAP lesions, ICG angiography typically reveals a focal area of intense hyperfluorescence that represents the neovascularization and corresponding late leakage within the retina from the intraretinal new vessels. Intraretinal exudates around the neovascularization stain with ICG in the mid-late phases, and at times, a retinal-retinal anastomosis can be visualized (108). Characteristic ICG findings are also seen in PCV that may distinguish it from occult CNV or RAP. Its use in evaluating CNV lesions and characterizing their natural history and responses to treatment have not been evaluated in large-scale clinical trials, but most feel it is valuable, particularly for the aforementioned disease states.

The development of OCT has greatly expanded our understanding of the anatomy, pathophysiology, natural history, and response to treatment of CNV. It demonstrates the cross-sectional anatomy of

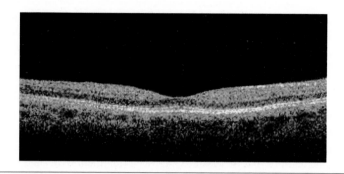

Figure 17. Normal OCT.

the inner retina, outer retina, Bruch's membrane, and choroid, and the pathologic states within each (Fig. 17). It allows for the quantitative measurement of intraretinal and subretinal fluid, and a three-dimensional assessment of volume of fluid is now calculable. Changes in these anatomic features allow the treating physician to easily and rapidly monitor responses to therapies such as intravitreal anti-VEGF injections and PDT (Fig. 18). The use of OCT has dramatically increased in the past 2 to 3 years because of its ease of use and sensitivity. In the future, OCT improvements will continue to enhance our understanding of macular and submacular pathology. Newer generations of OCT scanners provide unparalleled improvements in resolution to the level of ≤5 μm. Techniques employing confocal laser scanning systems, including those using adaptive optics technology, continue to enhance our abilities to visualize and understand macular disease.

From accurate clinical examination to supplemental imaging techniques, the treating physician comes to understand the pathoanatomy and pathophysiology of the disease process. This allows for the decisions to be made as to whether treatment is possible and/or which treatment regimen to pursue.

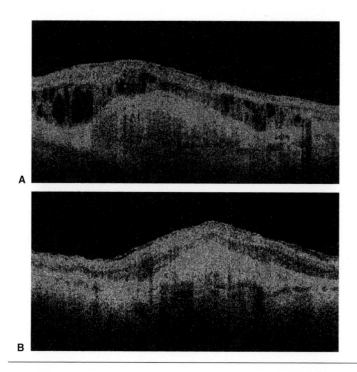

Figure 18. **A.** OCT of subfoveal CNV prior to intravitreal ranibizumab injection; note increased retinal thickness, subretinal elevation, and intraretinal edema. **B.** OCT of subfoveal CNV taken 4 weeks after 1 intravitreal ranibizumab injection; note decreased retinal thickness, subretinal elevation, and intraretinal edema.

Treatment of Neovascular AMD

George A. Williams

Laser Photocoagulation

During the 1980s and early 1990s, the Macular Photocoagulation Study Group demonstrated that thermal ablation of well-defined, small choroidal neovascular membranes is beneficial compared to the untreated natural history in select patients in a series of clinical trials (109–117). Thermal laser ablation is a fluorescein angiography directed procedure in which the location and type of neovascularization is determined by fluorescein angiographic characteristics. The treatment technique involves placement of high intensity retinal burns to the choroidal neovascular lesion with a green or red wavelength laser. The treatment endpoint is a confluent, white retinal burn with ablation of the underlying neovascular lesion. High laser powers and long pulse durations of up to 1 second are required. The study investigators emphasized the importance of ablating the entire neovascular lesion. This technique was used for extrafoveal, juxtafoveal, and subfoveal lesions.

In all of the studies, relatively small (<3.5 DA) lesions were evaluated. Such lesions probably represent less than 10% of the lesions comprising neovascular AMD and therefore, the utility of laser photocoagulation is low (118,119). The clinical endpoint in all of these studies was the rate of losing six or more Early Treatment Diabetic Retinopathy Study (ETDRS) lines of vision compared with untreated controls. This endpoint represents severe visual loss. The possibility of visual improvement with laser treatment was considered to be remote.

For juxtafoveal lesions, 5-year follow-up demonstrated a risk reduction (RR) of 1.82 for six lines of visual loss only for normotensive persons. Hypertensive persons did no better than untreated controls. Furthermore, the presence of occult CNV negated any benefit in all subjects (109–117). Recurrence of the neovascularization occurred in more than 50% of subjects (110,115). Thus, thermal laser for juxtafoveal lesions is rarely performed today.

For extrafoveal lesions, 5-year follow-up demonstrated an average loss of 5.2 lines compared with 7.1 lines of visual acuity in treated and control eyes, respectively (109). Recurrent neovascularization occurred in 54% of treated eyes with most occurring in the first year. However, for persons who did not experience a recurrence, the average visual acuity at 3 years was 20/50 (111).

For subfoveal lesions, the treatment effect of laser was related to initial lesion size and initial visual acuity. Eyes with small lesions (≤1 DA) and moderate or poor visual acuity (≤20/125) or medium lesions (>1≤2 DA) and poor visual acuity had the best visual outcome compared with controls. However, all of these eyes lost vision with treatment. Eyes with small lesions and visual acuity ≥20/100 or medium lesions with visual acuity ≥20/160 experienced more visual loss than untreated controls for the first 12 months after treatment and had some treatment benefit thereafter. Eyes with a large lesion (>2 DA) and visual acuity ≤20/200 had a treatment benefit throughout 4 years of follow-up. Eyes with large lesions and ≥20/160 vision did substantially worse than untreated controls for the first 18 months after treatment (112–114,116). Although the MPS demonstrated a statistically significant benefit in terms of the primary endpoint of less than six lines of visual loss, many retina specialists felt this difference was not clinically beneficial for most patients since most patients noticed immediate loss of vision following treatment. Therefore, the technique never gained widespread acceptance and is no longer used.

The above MPS trials clearly demonstrate that laser ablation is a suboptimal treatment for neovascular AMD with little potential for visual improvement. For the most part, MPS style laser treatment has been abandoned as a treatment for neovascular AMD with the possible exception of well-defined extrafoveal lesions.

Photodynamic Therapy

In 2000, the Food and Drug Administration (FDA) approved verteporfin with photodynamic therapy (PDT) for predominantly classic subfoveal lesions associated with AMD. In 2004, the Centers for Medicare and Medicaid Services (CMS) expanded coverage of PDT to include occult and minimally classic lesions that are ≤ 4 DA in size and associated with evidence of disease progression within 3 months. Disease progression is defined as loss of at least five letters on a standard eye chart, lesion growth of at least 1 DA, or the appearance of subretinal blood.

Photodynamic therapy is a two-step process involving, first, an intravenous infusion of verteporfin at a dose of 6 mg per M^2 of body surface area over 10 minutes followed by irradiance with a 689 nm laser for 83 seconds beginning 5 minutes after completion of the infusion delivering a total energy of 50 J/cm^2 at an intensity of 600 mW/cm^2 (600 mW/cm^2 x 83 seconds = 50 J/cm^2) (120). Verteporfin binds to low density lipoproteins (LDL) in the plasma during the infusion, which are then preferentially bound by choroidal neovascular tissue which express LDL receptors. Irradiation of the neovascular lesion by the laser creates toxic oxygen species that induce thrombosis and closure of the choroidal neovascularization. Although the thrombosis occurs predominantly in the choroidal neovascularization, there is evidence of some damage to both the choriocapillaris and RPE (121). Verteporfin is a potent photosensitizer, and patients must avoid direct sunlight or bright light exposure for a minimum of 24 hours after treatment. The FDA label recommends 5 days, but there is no data to support this. Like thermal laser, PDT is directed by fluorescein angiography characteristics. The size of the laser spot is determined by the greatest linear dimension (GLD) of the neovascular lesion measured on a fluorescein angiogram plus a 1,000 micron margin to assure the entire lesion is irradiated. Post-treatment, there is typically a hypofluorescent zone corresponding to the laser spot size signifying closure of the neovascularization. In the first few hours and days after PDT, there is often retinal edema, which can be seen on ocular coherence tomography (OCT) (122). This edema is probably due to VEGF, which is expressed after PDT (121). The thrombotic effect of PDT is short lived, and typically within 10 to 14 weeks there is reperfusion of the neovascular lesion. Evidence of leakage on FA is the indication for retreatment. Over 1 to 2 years of treatment, the frequency of leakage, and therefore treatment, typically decreases. Patients are usually followed on an every-3-month schedule for the first 1 to 2 years.

The first clinical trial to demonstrate the efficacy of PDT was Treatment of Age-Related Macular Degeneration with Photodynamic Therapy (TAP) Study, which studied classic subfoveal AMD lesions (120). Inclusion criteria were visual acuity of approximately 20/40 to 20/200 and a lesion size of ≤5,400 microns. The primary endpoint was the loss of less than 15 letters or 3 lines on the ETDRS chart, which was defined as moderate visual loss. After both 1 and 2 years of follow-up, treated eyes suffered less visual loss than controls; 39% vs. 54% and 57% vs. 62%, at 1 and 2 years, respectively. Subgroup analysis demonstrated that lesion composition was important. Predominantly classic lesions had a strong beneficial effect at 1 and 2 years. Minimally classic lesions, however, did not benefit. Treated eyes received an average of 3.4 treatments the first year, 2.2 treatments the second year, and 1.3 in the third year (123–125). An open label extension of the TAP Study demonstrated that these treatment benefits are maintained for up to 36 months (126).

The Verteporfin Photodynamic Therapy (VIP) study examined lesions with either occult with no classic CNV or classic CNV with baseline vision of 20/40 or better (127). The same moderate visual loss endpoint was used. At 1 year, there was no benefit in the primary endpoint compared with controls for all lesions. By 2 years, there was a benefit. Subgroup analysis demonstrated that for occult with no classic lesions the treatment benefit was greater for smaller lesions (≤ 4 DA) or lower levels of visual acuity (less than approximately 20/50). Subsequent retrospective subgroup analysis demonstrated that lesion size was also important for minimally classic lesions with a benefit seen in smaller lesions (< 4 DA) (128).

The Verteporfin in minimally classic CNV (VIM) Study examined the effects of both reduced fluence (300 mW/cm^2) and standard fluence (600 mW/ cm^2) in minimally classic lesions less than or equal to 6 DA in size. This study suggested the reduced fluence may be beneficial in such lesions and has led to ongoing trials examining reduced fluence (132).

The safety profile of PDT shows it is well tolerated. Ocular adverse events are most commonly transient, subjective visual disturbances that occur in up to 42% of patients in the first week following treatment. A less frequent but more serious adverse event is acute, severe visual acuity decrease, which is defined as a loss of ≥ 20 letters within 7 days of treatment. This occurred in 0.79% of subjects in the TAP study and 4.4% of subjects in the VIP Study. It is more common in large (> 4 DA) occult lesions and in eyes with good ($\geq 20/50$) vision. Visual acuity may improve over time to some degree in most patients (133). Systemic adverse events include injection site reactions (13.9%), photosensitivity reactions (2%), and infusion-related back pain (2%). The back pain typically resolves with discontinuation of drug infusion. It is recommended that if patients receive at least one half of the calculated dose, they receive laser treatment.

PDT was the first treatment for subfoveal CNV to be of clinical benefit in most patients with subfoveal neovascular AMD. Although it effectively slows the rate of visual loss and is generally well-tolerated, it rarely (<10%) results in significant visual improvement defined as a gain of three or more lines. At present, it is rarely used as monotherapy for neovascular AMD. However, because of its extended dosing schedule (every 3 months) and its anatomic effects on retarding lesion growth, there is increasing interest in PDT as a component of combination therapy which will be discussed later.

Surgery for Neovascular AMD

A variety of surgical techniques have been described and studied for the treatment of neovascular AMD involving submacular surgery and macular translocation (134). The rationale of submacular surgery is to remove the entire neovascular lesion with preservation of the overlying photoreceptors. The rationale of macular translocation is to displace the macula away from the neovascular lesion and into an area of normal RPE function. This then allows for thermal ablation of the neovascular lesion without damaging the macula. Only submacular surgery has been studied in large, multicenter randomized clinical trials.

Submacular surgery was first described in the late 1980s in several small case series which suggested clinical benefit. This apparent benefit was supported by a pilot study which led to the Submacular Surgery Trials (SST). For AMD, two groups of patients were studied. Group N had new subfoveal CNV (<9 DA) with evidence of classic CNV but no prior treatment (135). Group B had predominantly hemorrhagic subfoveal lesions defined as subretinal blood comprising more than 50% of the entire lesion (136).

In Group N, the surgical goal was complete removal of the neovascular complex by vitrectomy, subretinal dissection, and extraction of the lesion. The primary endpoint was a loss of two or more lines. Unfortunately, the SST demonstrated no difference between treatment and control eyes. Therefore, surgery as performed in the SST is not recommended for eyes similar to those enrolled in the SST Group N trial (135).

The eyes in Group B constituted a group with a particularly poor prognosis. The inclusion criteria were vision ≤20/100 to LP, ≥3.5 DA size lesion with 75% of the lesion posterior to equator and ≥50% of the lesion comprised of subretinal blood. Thus, a wide spectrum of hemorrhagic lesions was studied. The surgical goal was complete removal of subfoveal blood and any apparent neovascular lesion. At baseline, the median lesion size was 12 to 16 DA in both the treatment and observation cohorts, and median vision was 20/250 and 20/200 in treatment and observation cohorts, respectively. The study concluded that submacular surgery as performed in the SST did not increase the proportion of eyes with stabilized or improved visual acuity compared with observation. However, the surgery cohort had a decreased risk of losing six or more lines, and there was a twofold increase in vitreous hemorrhage in the observation cohort. There were significant complications in the surgery cohort including a 16% risk of rhegmatogenous retinal detachment and a sixfold increase in the need for cataract surgery. The SST concluded that surgery, as performed in the trial, is not recommended for similar lesions with visual acuity of 20/200 or worse. Surgery may be considered for similar lesions with visual acuity better than 20/200 with the caution that visual improvement is unlikely and there is significant risk of cataract and retinal detachment (136).

Another technique for the management of subretinal hemorrhage involves displacement of the subretinal blood utilizing an air or gas bubble and positioning. This technique can be performed with an intravitreal gas injection in the office or in conjunction with vitrectomy. Intravitreal or subretinal injection of tissue plasminogen activator is often used to try and lyse any clotted subretinal blood, thereby facilitating the pneumatic displacement. Small case series demonstrate that although the subretinal blood can be displaced in some patients, visual recovery is often limited (134,137,138).

Two macular translocation techniques have been described: limited and 360 degree (134,139,140). In limited translocation, a total retinal detachment is created by subretinal infusion after a complete vitrectomy (141,142). The sclera is then shortened by infolding or outfolding to create a relative excess of retinal surface area compared with the scleral surface area. The retina is then displaced, usually inferiorly, with a partial fluid-air exchange and positioning to move the macula away from the neovascular lesion, which is then ablated with laser postoperatively. In one case series, a mean translocation distance of 1,576 microns (range, 200 to 3,400 microns) was obtained, which limits this technique to relatively small lesions (142). About 50% of patients achieve adequate translocation for laser treatment and, of these, about 50% have recurrent SNV within one year. Overall, about 25% of patients are 20/80 at 1 year (141). Although initially promising, limited translocation has proven to be technically difficult and unpredictable and is no longer performed.

Total or 360 degree translocation is a surgical tour de force involving a complete vitrectomy, 360 degree peripheral retinotomy, creation of a total retinal detachment, removal of the neovascular lesion, retinal rotation around the optic nerve, retinal reattachment, silicone oil placement, and compensatory strabismus surgery to address the visual rotation (140,143–146). Small case series have demonstrated dramatic visual improvement in select patients. However, there is a steep learning curve with a significant intraoperative and postoperative complication rate. The technique is only performed in the better eye of patients with bilateral visual loss because of rotational distortion which prevents binocular vision. Currently, it is only performed at a few centers.

The concepts and techniques of surgery for neovascular AMD are undergoing continuing evolution. Transplantation of RPE and autologous repositioning of RPE, Bruch's membrane, and choriocapillaris have been described with limited success. However, the issues of transplant rejection and revascularization present formidable problems (147). At present, surgery is of little or no benefit for the vast majority of patients with neovascular AMD.

Feeder Vessel Technique

Feeder vessel treatment is based upon the visualization of select choroidal neovascular trunks that supply a neovascular lesion with high speed ICG angiography. Initial small case series reported clinical benefit in some patients (148). However, there are no randomized clinical trials to demonstrate either safety or efficacy, and this technique is confined to a few centers.

Combination Therapy

The term combination therapy describes the use of different therapies in combination for neovascular AMD. The concept of combination therapy is based upon an ever-improving understanding of the pathogenesis of neovascular AMD and the continuing development of new and often complementary treatment technologies. Choroidal neovascularization is a complex process, including multiple growth factors and cell types. Visual loss from CNV is multifactorial involving the effects of intraretinal edema, subretinal fluid, fibrovascular tissue, and inflammation on the photoreceptors RPE and choriocapillaris. Even within specific pathways such as the VEGF cascade, there are multiple redundancies that may circumvent a single therapeutic approach. Thus, there is a compelling rationale for a multiple target therapeutic approach.

The first combination therapy described was the combination of PDT and intravitreal triamcinolone acetonide (149,150). The rationale is that intravitreal triamcinolone may enhance the therapeutic efficacy and minimize the complications of PDT due to its anti-inflammatory and anti-permeability properties. Additionally, in contrast to anti-VEGF therapy, PDT limits CNV lesion growth (149,150). Several case series have demonstrated an apparent clinical benefit with combination therapy compared with PDT alone. Combination therapy has been reported to improve visual acuity and decrease the frequency of retreatment (149,151). These promising results have led to the formation of clinical trials which are ongoing to evaluate the benefits of PDT and intravitreal triamcinolone.

More recently, PDT has been combined with anti-VEGF agents including pegaptanib sodium, bevacizumab, and ranibizumab (149–153). The rationale is based on the fact that PDT increases VEGF expression shortly after treatment (121). Clinical trials are ongoing and will examine such issues as the dose, timing, and frequency of the injections as well as the fluence of the PDT. Additionally, a triple therapy combining PDT, intravitreal bevacizumab, and intravitreal dexamethasone has been reported to be beneficial (151). Some investigators are even revisiting thermal laser ablation for extrafoveal and juxtafoveal lesions in combination with anti-VEGF therapy. Although the rationale for combination therapy is compelling, and the preliminary results are promising, clinical trials are required to establish the safety and efficacy of this approach.

Anti-VEGF Therapy

Tarek S. Hassan

The management of AMD has taken a quantum leap forward with the development of anti-VEGF medications to treat active CNV. These drugs have allowed treating physicians to expect to preserve vision and, for the first time, aggressively seek visual improvement. The pathophysiology of neovascular AMD formation and the role of VEGF in this process have been discussed in earlier sections. In brief, the upregulation of VEGF caused by damage to Bruch's membrane begins a cascade of events: Binding of VEGF to VEGF receptors on endothelial cells → endothelial cell activation → production of cytokines that increase vascular permeability and lead to proliferation and migration of endothelial cells → formation of vascular buds and then tubules that develop into stabilized vessels with the growth of surrounding pericytes. Inhibition of the effects of VEGF on this process is felt to not only stabilize the anatomic pathology of CNV, and therefore visual acuity, but to lead to improvement in vision by reducing vascular hyperpermeability and resolving existing subretinal fluid and macular edema.

Anti-VEGF therapy may achieve its goals in one of three ways: (a) Block the effect of existing extracellular VEGF by binding it directly;

(b) Inhibit the response of the endothelial cell to VEGF; or (c) Inhibit the initial production of new VEGF. Methods that employ treatment strategies of each path are under investigation. Presently, the only mechanism by which any approved treatment acts is the binding and blocking of existing VEGF.

PEGAPTANIB SODIUM

The first proof of concept that anti-VEGF therapy was effective as treatment for CNV came from the VISION (VEGF Inhibition Study in Ocular Neovascularization) trials, from which positive outcomes led to FDA approval of pegaptanib sodium for the treatment of predominantly classic, minimally classic, and occult CNV in December 2004 (154).

Pegaptanib sodium (manufactured by Eyetech Pharmaceuticals as Macugen®) is a chemically synthesized 28-nucleotide ribonucleic acid aptamer that sensitively binds to extracellular VEGF-A isoforms of 165 or more amino acids in length. As an aptamer, pegaptanib acts like an antibody with high target specificity but is nonimmunogenic. It is the first aptamer therapeutically applied in humans. Its target, VEGF-165, is thought to be the major pathologic isoform of VEGF, and the efficiency of pegaptanib in blocking its effects was demonstrated in vivo and in vitro prior to clinical trials (155).

The VISION study began in 2001, consisting of two randomized, double-blinded, placebo-controlled clinical trials that included 117 centers worldwide and enrolled 1,186 patients (154). Principle inclusion criteria included patient age over 50 years, baseline VA = 20/40 to 20/320, and subfoveal CNV of all angiographic subtypes ≤12 DA in size. For predominantly classic lesions, 50% of the total lesion was required to have active CNV. Minimally classic lesions were defined as those with <50% of a classic component. Eyes without predominantly classic CNV were required to have subretinal hemorrhage, lipid, or ≥3 lines of vision loss in the past 12 weeks to prevent the enrollment of end-stage fibrotic lesions. Patients were randomized to receive an intravitreal injection of pegaptanib (0.3 mg, 1 mg, or 3 mg) or a sham injection into the study eye every 6 weeks for 54 weeks. Treating physicians had the ability to treat with PDT at their discretion if they felt it necessary to control disease progression.

The primary efficacy endpoint was the percentage of eyes losing less than 15 letters of vision measured by standardized ETDRS methods. All doses of pegaptanib were more effective than sham injections in achieving this goal, and there was no statistical difference between the different doses (Fig. 19) (154). Therefore, the results of the 0.3 mg group were carried forward to drug approval. The percentage of patients losing <15 letters was 70% in those receiving the 0.3 mg dose vs. 55% in the control group. The results were similar for

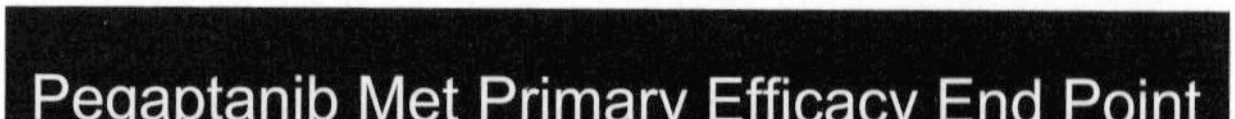

Pegaptanib Met Primary Efficacy End Point
% of Patients Losing <15 Letters at Week 54

	0.3 mg	1 mg	3 mg	Usual Care
	n=294	n=300	n=296	n=296
<15 letters (%)	70%	71%	65%	55%
P value	<.0001	.0003	.0310	--

27% relative increase in responders for 0.3-mg dose

Figure 19. VISION Trial Results: Eyes receiving pegaptanib meeting the primary study endpoint. From Gragoudas ES, et al. *N Engl J Med.* 2004; 351:2805–2816.

maintenance or gain of vision. Of those receiving pegaptanib, 11% gained 2 or more lines of vision compared with 6% of those receiving sham injections. Three or more lines of improved vision were seen in 6% of eyes receiving pegaptanib. The treatment benefits with pegaptanib were seen across all patient demographics. No association was found between treatment effect and lesion size, angiographic subtype, baseline vision, gender, or race. Re-randomization occurred at 54 weeks for 1,024 patients. Of those receiving pegaptanib from week 0 to week 102, 59% lost <15 letters compared with 45% of control eyes. The rate of vision loss was slowed by pegaptanib, but both the drug-treated group and control group lost vision overall (Fig. 20). The absolute difference in visual response between the treated and control eyes was ultimately somewhat disappointing to the retinal community and patients.

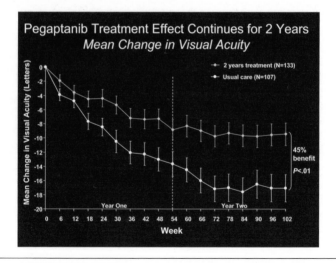

Figure 20. VISION Trial Results: Mean change of visual acuity over 2 years. From Gragoudas ES, et al. *N Engl J Med.* 2004; 351:2805–2816.

An unplanned retrospective subgroup analysis of the 54 week VI-SION data examined the response to treatment of eyes with *early lesions*–defined as those with small lesions (<2 DA), relatively good VA (≥54 letters), no prior PDT or thermal laser, and no scar or RPE atrophy within the lesion. It demonstrated that early lesions responded better to pegaptanib therapy than older lesions. In the eyes of the early treatment groups, 76% and 80% lost <15 letters compared with 50% and 57% in the respective sham groups. Severe vision loss was 10 times more likely in the sham group than the early treated groups. Visual improvement of ≥15 letters was noted in 12% and 20% of eyes compared with 4% and 0% in the sham groups (Fig. 21, 22) (156). Examples of successful treatment of CNV with pegaptanib as primary monotherapy are seen in Figures 23 and 24.

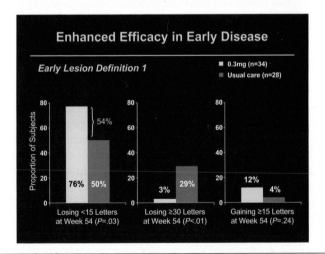

Figure 21. VISION Trial Subgroup Analysis: Enhanced efficacy in early lesion eyes (definition 1). From VISION Trial Group. *Retina.* 2005; 25: 815–827.

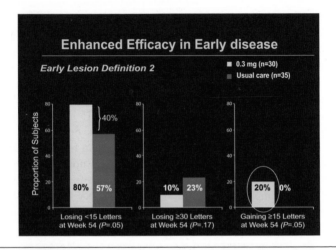

Figure 22. VISION Trial Subgroup Analysis: Enhanced efficacy in early lesion eyes (definition 2). From VISION Trial Group. *Retina*. 2005; 25: 815–827.

No systemic safety issues were identified with pegaptanib. Ocular adverse events were seen at a low rate: retinal detachment in 0.6% of eyes and endophthalmitis in 1.3% After a protocol change increased attention to aseptic technique, the rate of endophthalmitis dropped from 0.18% to 0.03% per injection.

The VISION trial was the first study to confirm the role of VEGF in the pathogenesis of neovascular AMD and demonstrate the efficacy of blocking VEGF in the treatment of CNV. Its treatment effect was modest and was most effective in slowing eventual vision loss. Its use, however, was a major step forward in the treatment of AMD, and although its performance in improving vision was generally disappointing, it forcefully opened the door for the greater success of later anti-VEGF agents such as bevacizumab and ranibizumab.

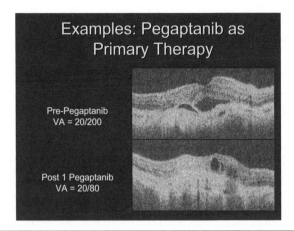

Figure 23. Example of pegaptanib therapy: VA improvement with substantial clearing of intraretinal and subretinal fluid shown by OCT.

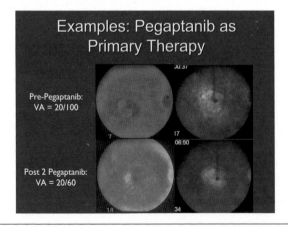

Figure 24. Example of pegaptanib therapy: VA improvement and FA demonstration of reduced vascular activity following one intravitreal injection.

Anti-VEGF Antibodies: Ranibizumab & Bevacizumab

In order to block VEGF activity that promotes neovascular AMD, researchers developed monoclonal antibodies to target VEGF directly under the retina. Starting with a full-length mouse monoclonal antibody that they synthesized, researchers at Genentech, Inc. altered its structure to create a drug with properties optimized for use as a treatment for CNV. At roughly the same time they were altering the parent antibody in other ways to create chemotherapeutic drugs for systemic cancer treatment. In the early-mid 1990s, they elected to take two distinct developmental paths to achieve these goals: (a) Humanize the entire full-length antibody to have systemic chemotherapeutic activity, and (b) Humanize and affinity mature only one of the binding portions of the molecule to act specifically in the target tissue of the eye as an AMD treatment. They felt that a smaller molecule would better penetrate to the subretinal space, cause less local inflammation, and have little or no systemic penetration or toxicity. Thus, two distinct parallel developmental tracks were put in place: One for the larger full antibody (bevacizumab) for colon cancer treatment and one for the much smaller antibody fragment (ranibizumab) for AMD therapy (157–159).

Ranibizumab

Ranibizumab (formerly known as rhuFab V2), developed by Genentech, Inc. as Lucentis®, is a small antibody fragment synthesized to have a 100 times increased affinity for all isoforms of VEGF-A, in contrast to pegaptanib which only blocks VEGF-A$_{165}$. It has been shown to be effective at reducing vascular permeability and angiogenesis in vitro and in vivo (Fig.25), as well as in an experimental model of laser-induced CNV following intraocular injection (160). Experimental evaluation has demonstrated that after intravitreal

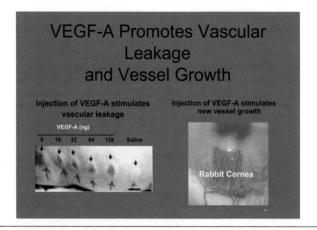

Figure 25. VEGF stimulates vascular leakage in a Miles Assay (blue dye from the mouse circulation leaks from intradermal VEGF injection sites)–left; VEGF stimulates new vessel growth in a rabbit model of corneal neovascularization–right. Adapted from Murohara T, et al. Vascular Endothelial Growth Factor/Vascular Permeability Via Nitric Oxide and Prostacyclin. *Circulation* 1998;97:99–107.

injection, it is rapidly distributed to the retina in 6 to 24 hours and has a terminal half-life of 3 days (161).

Clinical Trials

Convincing early safety and efficacy data were seen following frequent multiple intravitreal injections of ranibizumab in phase I/II clinical trials (162–164). These led to the two pivotal phase III clinical trials–MARINA (Minimally Classic/Occult Trial of the Anti-VEGF Antibody Ranibizumab in the Treatment of Neovascular AMD) and ANCHOR (Anti-VEGF Antibody for the Treatment of Predominantly Classic Choroidal Neovascularization in AMD)

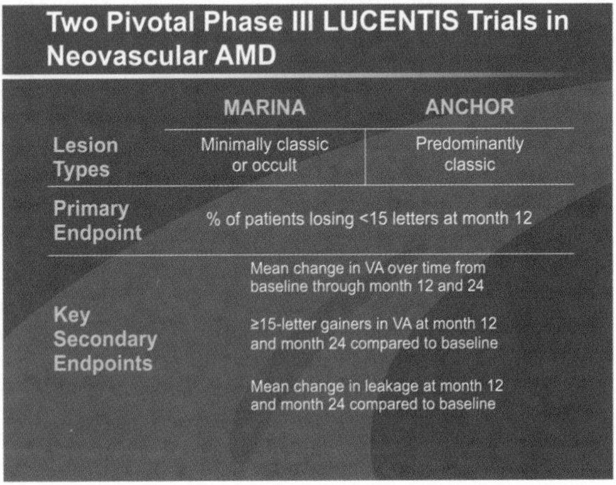

Figure 26. Key characteristics of the two pivotal phase III ranibizumab trials – MARINA and ANCHOR.

(165,166)–whose data ultimately led to the FDA approval of ranibizumab in June 2006 for the treatment of all forms of neovascular AMD (Fig. 26).

MARINA

This randomized, multicenter, double-blinded, parallel group, placebo-controlled trial evaluated the intravitreal injection of 0.3 mg and 0.5 mg of ranibizumab vs. sham injection in 716 patients with minimally classic or pure occult subfoveal CNV with recent disease progression (Fig. 27). Entry criteria included age ≤50 years, best corrected vision between 20/40 and 20/320, no prior PDT or laser, and evidence of blood or lesion growth by FA or decreased vision. Patients received an injection of either dose of ranibizumab or a sham injection monthly for 1 year. PDT was allowed if significant vision loss oc-

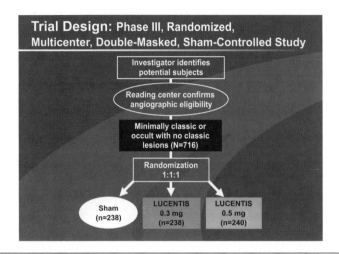

Figure 27. MARINA Trial design.

curred or the lesion converted to a predominantly classic configuration. The groups were randomized 1:1:1; baseline characteristics were similar among the groups (165,166).

At 12 months, 95% of patients treated with 0.5 mg ranibizumab lost ≤15 letters compared with 62% that received sham treatment. Vision improved by ≥15 letters in 34% of patients receiving ranibizumab vs. roughly 5% of placebo eyes. Vision of 20/40 or better was obtained in 40% of ranibizumab eyes compared with 11% of sham eyes (165). The benefits of the drug were maintained at the end of year 2, with a mean letter difference between the treated and control group of 21.5 ETDRS letters–the treatment group having gained an average of 6.6 letters (Figs. 28–30). The visual improvements were gradual and progressive through the 2 years of treatment as demonstrated in Figure 31 that illustrates the time to the first gain of ≥15 letters of acuity. At

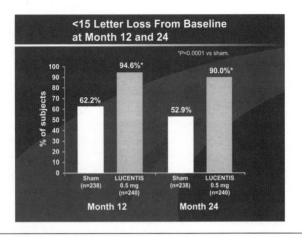

Figure 28. MARINA Results: <15 letter loss, months 12 and 24.

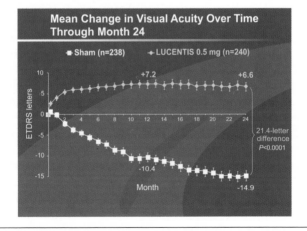

Figure 29. MARINA Results: Mean VA change through month 24.

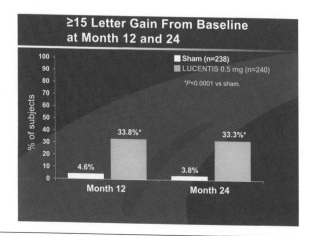

Figure 30. MARINA Results: ≥15 letter gain at months 12 and 24.

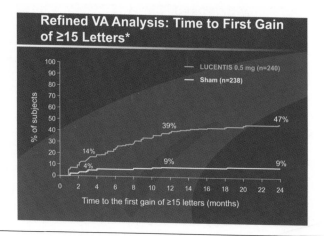

Figure 31. MARINA Results: Kaplan-Meier analysis illustrating the time to the first gain of ≥15 letters.

year 2, 90% of treated eyes lost <15 letters from baseline compared with 53% of sham eyes. At baseline, 15% of both sham and treatment group eyes had vision ≥20/40; by year 2, 42% of treated eyes achieved vision of ≥20/40 versus 6% of sham eyes. The benefits of ranibizumab were seen in all subgroups, regardless of lesion size, visual acuity, or lesion type. Several predetermined anatomic outcomes were assessed in MARINA. At 12 months, the mean area of leakage or stain at 12 months was less in ranibizumab eyes than control eyes, decreasing from 3.5 DA to 1.6 DA in treated eyes vs. increasing from 3.5 DA to 4.7 DA in the control eyes. By 24 months, the mean area of leakage in the treated eyes had continued to decrease to 1.3 DA. The differences between the sham and treated eyes were maintained at 2 years (Fig. 32). At 12 months, the treated eyes had an increase in the percentage

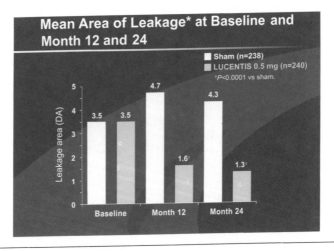

Figure 32. MARINA Results: Mean area of CNV leakage, baseline vs. 12 and 24 months.

of patients showing no FA leakage from 5% at baseline to 42%, whereas the sham group showed only a mild increase from 5% to 11%. The mean total lesion size stayed constant from 4.5 DA at baseline to 4.6 DA over 12 months in the treated group but increased from 4.4 DA at baseline to 6.7 DA at 1 year in the sham group. In treated eyes, the mean foveal thickness measured by OCT improved from 327 μm at baseline to 204 μm at 12 months, but in the control eyes, it remained largely unchanged over this period (167).

Subgroup analysis of the MARINA data at 24 months demonstrated that the percentage of patients losing less than 15 letters and the percentage of patients gaining ≥15 letters was equivalent across all ranges of presenting baseline vision except for 20/50 or better eyes for which there was significantly less fluctuation either way given the good presenting vision. Similarly, the percentage of eyes losing <15 letters and those gaining ≥15 letters was equivalent regardless of the CNV size at presentation. A Kaplan-Meier analysis of visual improvements over the 24-month follow-up looked at the time taken to obtain ≥15 letters visual improvement for the first time. At 3 months, it was seen in 14% of treated eyes and 4% of sham eyes; at 12 months, it was seen in 39% of treated eyes compared with 9% of sham eyes; and at 24 months, it was seen in 47% of treated eyes and 9% of sham eyes. This data demonstrates the progressive improvement in vision that occurs from the first month through the 24 months of follow-up. Visual improvements obtained by 12 months were maintained over the next 12 months of follow-up (167). A representative example of outcomes with ranibizumab therapy from the MARINA trial is shown in Figures 33–35.

No increased serious systemic adverse events were seen in the treated group. Serious ocular adverse events that occurred more commonly in the treated than control group were uveitis and endophthalmitis, occurring <1% of the time.

The 1-year MARINA data were presented at the 2005 American Society of Retina Specialists (ASRS) Annual Meeting surrounded by

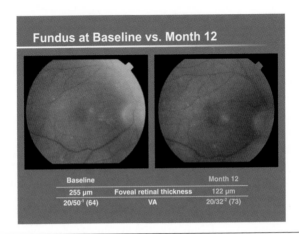

Figure 33. MARINA Examples: Fundus photos–baseline vs. month 12 outcome; decreased foveal thickness, improved VA.

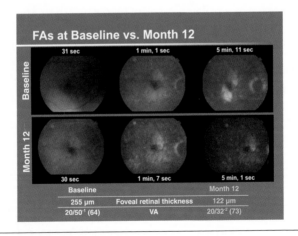

Figure 34. MARINA Examples: Fluorescein angiography–baseline vs. month 12 outcome; decreased fluorescein leakage.

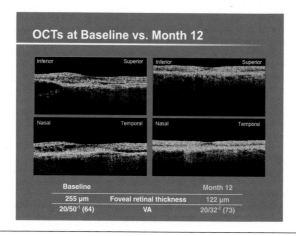

Figure 35. AMARINA Examples: OCT–baseline vs. month 12 outcome; decreased foveal thickness, decreased intraretinal edema.

a great deal of excitement among physicians, medical paraprofessionals, industry representatives, financial analysts, and most importantly, patients, as they represented the first evidence that wide-scale visual improvement and a remarkable level of visual stability could be achieved following the treatment of neovascular AMD. A new paradigm in the treatment of AMD had been ushered into the ophthalmologic world. The 2-year MARINA data demonstrating consistency in the excellent visual outcomes only strengthened the evolving sentiment that ranibizumab had fundamentally changed our approach to AMD.

Anchor

This phase III trial was a two-year randomized, multicenter, double-masked trial in which 423 patients were randomly assigned in a 1:1:1 ratio to receive a monthly intravitreal injection of either 0.3 mg or 0.5 mg of ranibizumab and a sham PDT treatment at baseline or monthly sham injections, a PDT treatment at baseline, and quarterly PDT treatments as necessary (Fig. 36). Entry criteria included age ≥50 years old, vision of 20/40 to 20/320, a predominantly classic subfoveal lesion ≤5,400 μm in greatest linear dimension, no prior treatment, and no significant foveal scarring. After one year, 96% of eyes receiving 0.5 mg of ranibizumab lost fewer than 15 letters of vision compared with 64% of eyes in the sham (PDT) group. Visual improvement of ≥15 letters was seen in 40% of those in the 0.5 mg ranibizumab group compared with 6% in the sham (PDT) group. Mean visual improvement was 11.3 letters in the treated group vs. a mean visual decrease of 9.5 letters in the sham group (Figs. 37–39). The time to first gain of ≥15 letters is shown in Figure 40. Anatomic outcomes were superior with ranibizumab in ANCHOR. The area of classic CNV increased until month 6 before stabilizing in the PDT group, whereas it decreased at month 3 and at month 6 prior to stabi-

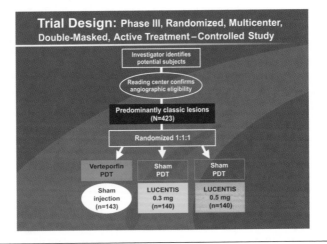

Figure 36. ANCHOR: Trial design.

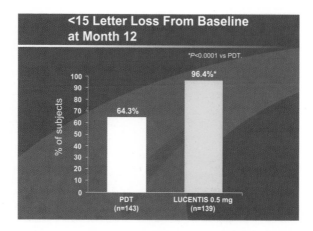

Figure 37. ANCHOR Results: <15 letter loss, month 12.

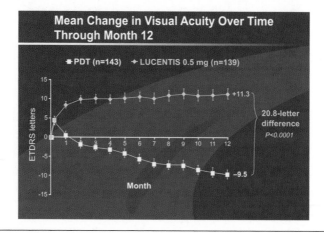

Figure 38. ANCHOR Results: Mean VA change through month 12.

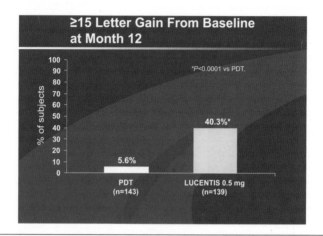

Figure 39. ANCHOR Results: ≥15 letter gain at month 12.

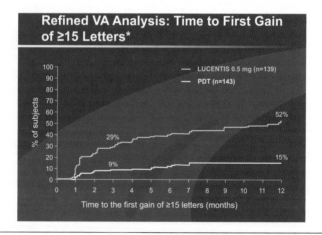

Figure 40. ANCHOR Results: Kaplan-Meier analysis illustrating the time to the first gain of ≥15 letters.

lizing in the treated group. The area of leakage increased from approximately 3 DA to 3.4 DA by month 12 in the PDT group but decreased from approximately 3 DA to 0.87 DA in the 0.5 mg ranibizumab group (Fig. 41). By month 12, no leakage was seen in 42% of eyes receiving 0.5 mg ranibizumab compared with 8% of PDT eyes. Mean total lesion size remained stable in the treated eyes but increased significantly and consistently over the 12-month follow-up period in those in the sham (PDT) group. Mean foveal thickness was decreased in both groups but more significantly in the ranibizumab treated eyes (402 → 307 μm vs. 399 → 210 μm). Recent subgroup analysis of the ANCHOR data revealed the superiority of ranibizumab over PDT regardless of vision at baseline, lesion size, presence of occult component within the CNV, or other patient characteristics. The time to first gain of ≥3 lines of vision was evaluated

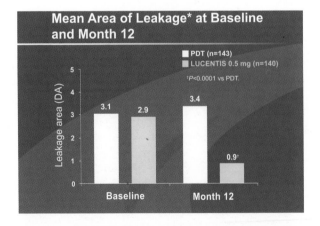

Figure 41. ANCHOR Results: Mean area of CNV leakage, baseline vs. 12 months.

by further subgroup analysis using Kaplan-Meier statistical methods. By 3 months, 29% of treated eyes had gained ≥3 lines of vision versus 9% of sham (PDT) eyes; by 12 months, 52% of treated eyes had gained ≥3 lines of vision compared with 15% of sham (PDT) eyes (168). A representative example of the response to ranibizumab seen in the ANCHOR trial is shown in Figures 42–44. Ocular side effects were inflammation in 11% and endophthalmitis in 1%. No significant differences in systemic side effects were noted.

Pooled data from both MARINA and ANCHOR demonstrated no statistically significant difference in either ocular or systemic side effects between ranibizumab treated eyes and control eyes. The only imbalance suggested was a slight increase in the number of arterial thromboembolic events, as described by the Antiplatelet Trialists' Collaboration (APTC), in those receiving 0.5 mg ranibizumab (2.1% vs. 1.1%). The clinical significance of this imbalance is unclear at this

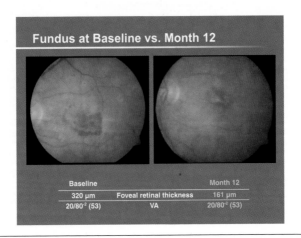

Figure 42. ANCHOR Examples: Fundus photos – baseline vs. month 12 outcome; decreased foveal thickness, stable VA.

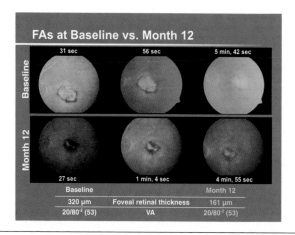

Figure 43. ANCHOR Examples: Fluorescein angiography – baseline vs. month 12 outcome; decreased fluorescein leakage and lesion size.

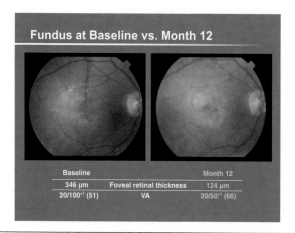

Figure 44. ANCHOR Examples: OCT – baseline vs. month 12 outcome; decreased foveal thickness, decreased subretinal fluid.

point, particularly given that since FDA approval of ranibizumab, no reports of increased rates of systemic abnormalities have surfaced. The pretreatment incidence of immunoreactivity was 0% to 3% among all groups receiving ranibizumab in both phase III trials. After 12 to 24 months, the incidence of low antibody titers was seen in roughly 1% to 6% of patients. The clinical significance of this finding has yet to be determined, although some of the eyes with the highest antibody titers demonstrated uveitis after injection.

Other Trials

Focus (169) A randomized, single-masked, placebo-controlled, multicenter trial comparing ranibizumab plus PDT vs. PDT alone in eyes with predominantly classic subfoveal CNV. Eligibility criteria were similar to that in ANCHOR except that prior PDT was allowed for inclusion. Patients were randomized 1:2 to PDT plus sham injection or PDT plus 0.5 mg ranibizumab injection and followed for 1 year. At month 12, 90% of ranibizumab and PDT eyes lost <15 letters vs. 68% of sham plus PDT eyes. Visual improvement of ≥15 letters was seen in 24% of treated eyes vs. 5% in the PDT alone arm; a difference of 13.1 letters existed between the 2 groups. No safety concerns other than increased intraocular inflammation were noted. This uveitis was attributed to a previous formulation of the drug not used in the phase III trials and not later commercialized.

Pier (167) Evaluated the effects on outcomes of a less frequent ranibizumab dosing schedule than employed in the phase III trials. Lesions of all subtypes were enrolled from 184 patients and randomized 1:1:1 to receive 0.5 mg ranibizumab, 0.3 mg ranibizumab, or sham injection, given once monthly for 3 doses and then every 3 months for a total of 12 and 24 months of follow-up. At 12 months, vision loss ≤15 letters was seen in 90% of eyes treated with 0.5 mg ranibizumab compared with 49% in the sham group. However, visual improvement of ≥15 letters was noted in only 13% of 0.5 mg ranibizumab treated eyes compared with 10% of sham eyes. Mean change of visual acuity in ETDRS letters was +4.3 in the 0.5 mg ranibizumab group and −8.7 in the sham group—a clinically significant difference (Figs. 45–47). The response of a representative eye from this trial is shown in Figures 48–50. Unfortunately, the magnitude of visual improvement with this dosing schedule was far inferior to that seen in the MARINA and ANCHOR trials, demonstrating that a firm quarterly dosing schedule is not nearly as efficacious of a treatment regimen as a firm monthly dosing schedule. Likely, the optimal dosing schedule is neither of these as patients and physicians seek to maximize visual outcomes and minimize the frequency of injections. Other trials have been, or are being, done to help clarify optimal treatment regimens.

Pronto (Prospective Ocular Coherence Tomography Imaging of Patients with Neovascular AMD Treated with Intra-Ocular

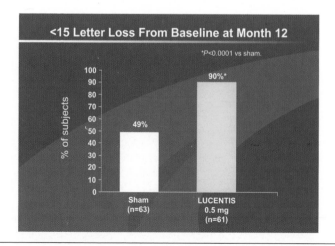

Figure 45. PIER Results: <15 letter loss, month 12.

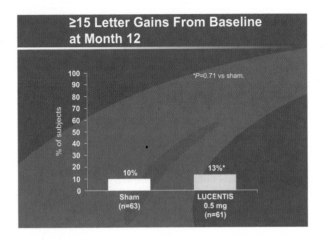

Figure 46. PIER Results: ≥15 letter gain at month 12.

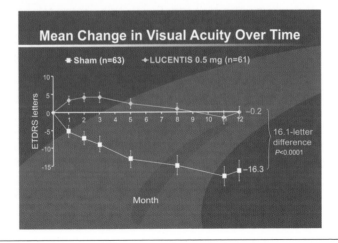

Figure 47. PIER Results: Mean VA change through month 12.

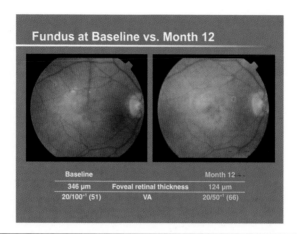

Figure 48. PIER Examples: Fundus photos – baseline vs. month 12 outcome; decreased foveal thickness, improved VA.

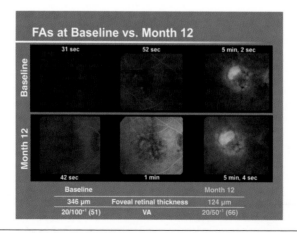

Figure 49. PIER Examples: Fluorescein angiography – baseline vs. month 12 outcome; decreased fluorescein leakage.

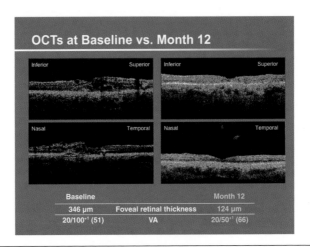

Figure 50. PIER Examples: OCT – baseline vs. month 12 outcome; decreased foveal thickness, decreased intraretinal edema.

Ranibizumab)–An investigator sponsored trial done at Bascom Palmer Eye Institute, University of Miami, headed by Phillip Rosenfeld, M.D., Ph.D. evaluated an alternative dosing strategy of ranibizumab. Forty patients with subfoveal CNV of all types, vision of 20/40 to 20/320, and potentially a history of prior CNV treatment, were treated with 3 consecutive monthly injections of 0.5 mg ranibizumab and then followed monthly by clinical examination, OCT, and FA to determine the need for retreatment. After the initial three injections, re-injection was done only if there was an increase in foveal thickness of ≥100 µm or residual subretinal fluid noted by OCT, vision loss of 5 letters with recurrent fluid seen on OCT, new classic CNV seen by FA, or new macular hemorrhage seen by examination or photography. In this trial, 57% of lesions were minimally classic, 25% pure occult, and 18% predominantly classic. A median of

5 injections was performed per subject and the median time to rein-
jection after the initial series was 3 months. Seven of the 40 patients
needed no further injections. By 12 months, the mean decrease in
foveal thickness was 180 μm, vision loss <15 letters was seen in 95%
of eyes, and visual improvement of ≥15 letters was seen in 35% of
eyes. No adverse effects were noted. This trial impressively demonstrated that this treatment and follow-up regimen may maintain the
gains seen in the phase III trials with fewer than monthly injections.

Sailor This is an ongoing trial that further explores the optimal
ranibizumab treatment regimen. This 1-year trial began in November
2005 with patients getting ranibizumab once monthly for 3 months
and then on an as-needed basis. It enrolled 5,000 patients who were
treated with either 0.3 mg or 0.5 mg of ranibizumab to determine the
best way to use this form of anti-VEGF therapy in the treatment of
neovascular AMD.

Ranibizumab: Post-FDA Approval

Since FDA approval, many thousands of ranibizumab injections have
been done in the U.S. for neovascular AMD. Anecdotal reports and
early case series suggest that the results reported in the phase III trials are seen in clinical practice by most treating physicians.
Refinements in injection technique, patient flow management, timing
of follow-up visits, and the use of diagnostic studies to determine
CNV activity have been made and continue to evolve as the retinal
community increasingly embraces intravitreal anti-VEGF therapy as
an integral part of their therapeutic practice. Examples of typically
good responses to ranibizumab treatment in several eyes are shown in
Figures 51–53.

Bevacizumab

As mentioned earlier, bevacizumab, a full-length humanized monoclonal anti-VEGF antibody is structurally related but distinctly dif-

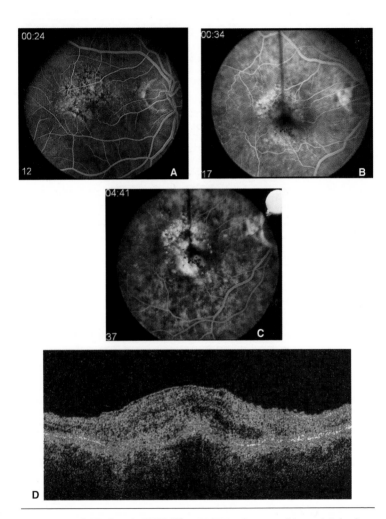

Figure 51. A–D. Occult CNV, VA = 20/200 prior to ranibizumab injection.

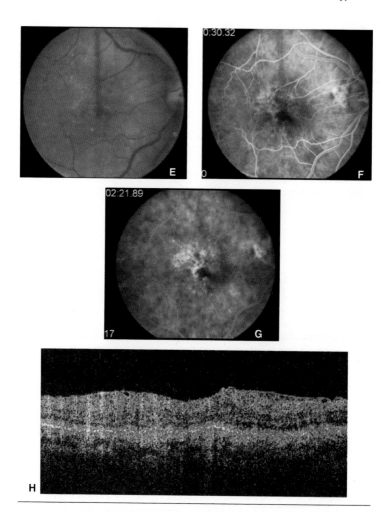

Figure 51. **E–H.** Occult CNV, VA = 20/70 after 3 ranibizumab injections.

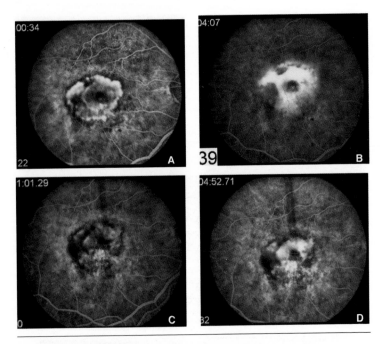

Figure 52. A–B. Classic CNV, VA = 20/400 prior to ranibizumab injection. **C–D.** Classic CNV, VA = 20/100 following 4 ranibizumab injections.

ferent from ranibizumab. Scientists at Genentech, Inc. developed it on a parallel track from the same progenitor molecule. Like ranibizumab, it binds all isoforms of VEGF-A, making it an excellent candidate to be used as an anti-angiogenic drug for a variety of conditions. It was developed and then approved by the FDA as a chemotherapeutic agent for colorectal cancer in 2004 as Avastin®. Shortly thereafter, it was tried as systemic therapy for neovascular AMD. The SANA (Systemic Bevacizumab [Avastin®] Therapy for Neovascular Age-Related Macular Degeneration) Trial, an open-label

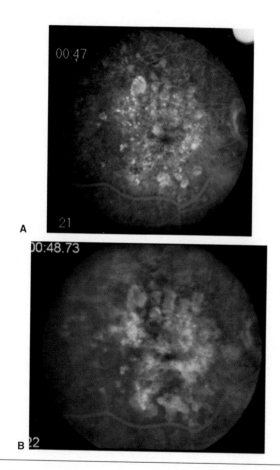

Figure 53. **A.** Occult CNV, VA = 20/200 prior to ranibizumab injection.
B. Occult CNV, VA = 20/100 following 3 ranibizumab injections.

single-center uncontrolled study evaluated eyes with subfoveal CNV and vision of 20/40 to 20/400 that were treated with 5 mg/kg intravenous infusion of bevacizumab and then retreated with 1 or 2 additional doses given at 2-week intervals. Data from 18 eyes showed visual improvement of 8 letters and a reduction of mean foveal thickness by 157 μm at week 1 and visual improvement of 13 letters with reduction of mean foveal thickness of 112 μm by week 24. The only adverse event noted was an elevation of systolic blood pressure, controlled with a change of medication (170). This series demonstrated that bevacizumab could successfully treat CNV, but the specter of systemic complications in elderly patients receiving frequent intravenous doses of this chemotherapeutic drug was raised when the elevated risk of thromboembolic events (4.4%) was seen in patients being treated with the drug for colorectal cancer. At the same time, investigators were observing good outcomes using the similar anti-VEGF agent ranibizumab delivered intravitreally in the Phase III clinical trials, and thus this led to the early intravitreal usage of bevacizumab.

The successful use of intravitreal bevacizumab injection to treat neovascular AMD was first reported in 2005 (171). The drug was shown to sufficiently penetrate the retina to reach the subretinal target tissue and exert an effect. Excitement about its potential use was fueled by its immediate availability to physicians for off-label use at a time when ranibizumab was potentially 1 year away from FDA approval for use outside of controlled trials—and by its low cost. Avery et al (172) reported their results using monthly intravitreal injections of 1.25 mg of bevacizumab in 81 eyes with CNV, most of which had been previously treated with PDT or pegaptanib, until macular edema or subretinal fluid resolved. Follow-up was from 4 to 15 weeks. Median vision improved from 20/200 at baseline to 20/80 by month 2, OCT-measured mean foveal thickness decreased, and no adverse events were reported. Spaide et al (173) reported similar outcomes in 266 eyes, 70% of which had received some prior treatment. Median vision improved from 20/184 at baseline to 20/137 at month 1,

20/122 at month 2, and 20/109 at month 3. Mean foveal thickness decreased as expected. Two eyes reportedly developed vitritis, but otherwise no other adverse events could be reliably linked to the drug. A prospective trial by Bashur et al (174) demonstrated that 3 monthly injections of 2.5 mg of bevacizumab in 17 eyes resulted in improved mean VA from 20/252 to 20/76 and decreased mean foveal thickness.

Humans receiving electroretinograms (ERGs) up to 4 weeks after single bevacizumab injection showed no photoreceptor toxicity (175), but the pharmacology, pharmacokinetics, and true toxicology following intravitreal administration remains poorly elucidated. Despite this, many thousands of intravitreal bevacizumab injections for neovascular AMD have been given worldwide. An internet-based survey database was developed to voluntarily track potential adverse events from 7,113 injections done in 5,228 patients from 12 countries. Fung et al (176) reported on the data at the annual ARVO meeting in May 2006. Severe ocular adverse events were very infrequently seen. Uveitis was noted in 0.14%, endophthalmitis in <0.1%, retinal detachment in <0.1%, cataract in 0.01%, central retinal artery occlusion in 0.02%, and acute vision loss in 0.07%. Potential linked systemic side effects included elevated blood pressure (0.221%), cerebrovascular accident (0.07%), transient ischemic attack (0.01%), and death (0.02%). This trial failed to demonstrate any significant elevation of adverse events that would prevent increasingly widespread usage of intravitreal bevacizumab.

Many questions currently surround the use of intravitreal bevacizumab in the absence of any large-scale controlled randomized clinical trial data that demonstrates its safety and efficacy. Yet because of the biochemical similarities between bevacizumab and ranibizumab and the widespread anecdotal data that reports good visual and anatomic outcomes with bevacizumab usage, there is the perception among many in the retinal community that the two drugs act equivalently. The excellent outcomes reported in the phase III ranibizumab trials have become expected by users of bevacizumab, and given the drug's low cost and ability to meet such expectations to date, bevacizumab continues to be widely used as an integral part of primary therapy of neovascular AMD. Some treating physicians use either bevacizumab or ranibizumab exclusively; some utilize each without clear distinction; some use bevacizumab with greater frequency in patients without adequate insurance coverage. As more experience is gained with ranibizumab, its use may increase, although if physicians do not see a significant advantage of this more expensive drug, they may gravitate towards using more bevacizumab. Ranibizumab is backed by the weight of excellent phase III prospective data while bevacizumab is backed by its price—1/50th to 1/100th that of ranibizumab.

The National Eye Institute of the National Institutes of Health has started a trial to compare the two drugs head-to-head in a randomized, multicenter, prospective, comparative trial. It will begin enrolling patients in early 2007 and expects to evaluate the efficacy of these drugs when used similarly in eyes matched by the same inclusion criteria. The public health value of this study cannot be overstated. It will likely provide information that will be integral in shaping the future direction of anti-VEGF therapy with the two most common drugs used for AMD.

Impact of Anti-VEGF Therapy on Quality of Life

Quality of life (QOL) assessments of treated macular degeneration patients provide an excellent objective look at the impact of both the disease and the therapeutic regimen on the ability of patients to perform basic activities of daily living and maintain some level of independent lifestyle. The MARINA and ANCHOR trials were the first large-scale AMD trials to collect such information and then use it to justify the widespread adoption of anti-VEGF therapy to improve the lives of patients.

The National Eye Institute Visual Function Questionnaire (NEI-VFQ 25) was administered in MARINA and ANCHOR at baseline and then at months 2, 3, 6, 9, and 12 (177). This instrument has 25 items divided into 11 different subscales: General health, general vision, near vision difficulties (reading normal newsprint, seeing well up close, finding objects on crowded shelf), distance vision difficulties (going out to movies or plays, going down stairs at night, reading street signs), dependency on others due to vision (needing much help from others, staying home most of the time, relying too much on others' word), peripheral vision limitations, color vision limitations, social functioning limitations due to vision (seeing how people react, visiting others), role limitations due to vision (accomplishing less, limited in endurance), driving difficulties (daylight familiar places, nighttime familiar places, difficult conditions), mental health symptoms due to vision (frustration, embarrassment, lack of control, worry), and ocular pain (amount of pain, amount of time with pain). Each subscale is given a score of 0 to 100, and an overall score is also generated. A 10-point change in QOL score over time is considered a meaningful change, either in the subscales or overall score (178). Ranibizumab treated eyes had higher mean NEI-VFQ 25 scores than controls at each follow-up visit in the 12 months after initiation of MARINA and ANCHOR. Significant differences between the treated and untreated eyes were visible as early as at 2 months. At 1 year, the treated eyes had a mean change from baseline that was 12–13 points higher than sham eyes in near activities in MARINA and 2.8–5.3 points higher in near activities in ANCHOR. Treated eyes had a 12.6–12.9 points greater than sham eyes in distance activity in MARINA and 4.7–7.6 points greater in distance activities in ANCHOR. They had an average of 8.4–11.5 points higher than sham in vision-specific dependency in MARINA and 9.6–10.4 points higher for the same parameters in ANCHOR. Higher scores in all predetermined activities were seen in the treated eyes, which were much more likely to have a 10+ point difference than sham eyes in all subscales and composite scores. Certainly these findings come as little surprise as they correlate well with the visual acuity improvement seen in these trials, although it is important to note that QOL assessments in AMD patients are more often a reflection of the functioning of the better seeing eye as subjects respond to questions about their abilities to perform tasks with the whole of their vision (179). Less than 50% of the study eyes in MARINA were the better of the subjects' eyes, and thus the changes seen in NEI-VFQ 25 scores obtained in these trials may underrepresent the QOL impact of improved vision from ranibizumab treatment.

Patient and Physician Expectations

The emergence of intravitreal anti-VEGF therapy has fundamentally changed the expectations of both physicians and patients as they look to the future in their struggles with neovascular AMD. Most now reasonably expect to at least avoid moderate or severe vision loss and reasonably hope to gain some vision after appropriate treatment regimens are carried out. Patients have greater access to information about ongoing research and trial results from television, radio, newspapers, internet, and even other patients, and may present for medical care armed with the intent to "get better" or "see well again." It thus becomes incumbent on the physician to take adequate time to explain the facts of the trial outcomes and relate these to the specific features of each individual patient. Many among the elderly are not used to understanding complicated treatment algorithms and expected outcomes and thus require a dedicated approach to manage these expectations. Patients may come to treatment expecting to have such visual improvement after ranibizumab that they may again drive, read, or become entirely independent when the anatomic dysfunction is known to not be able to allow such an outcome. Patients must realize that vision loss is possible, sometimes to a significant degree, even if they receive anti-VEGF therapy. Most patients, in fact, will not gain vision as the phase III trials indicate, and yet such is so often expected. Furthermore, patients must expect the rigors of the treatment regimen that may include many (≥ 12) intravitreal injections, along with numerous visits and/or imaging studies. Some patients may potentially require lifelong treatment—it is unknown from currently available data—and yet vision may be maintained with such aggressive continued care. Physicians should be armed with informational material to educate patients such that they can understand the processes involved, particularly given that the health literacy of many patients, particularly the elderly, may not be high and may decline with advancing age, debilitating health, and failing vision.

CURRENT INVESTIGATIONAL TREATMENTS

Beyond the striking advances in the treatment of neovascular AMD that have occurred over the last several years, culminating most recently with the approval and widespread use of bevacizumab and ranibizumab, there is a promising future for improved treatments as several other therapies are currently in development—either to be used as monotherapy or in combination with others.

Anti-VEGF Agents in Development

The monoclonal antibody ranibizumab was the first AMD treatment drug shown to significantly improve vision rather than simply reduce vision loss; it did so by inhibiting VEGF-A as described earlier. Drugs in various stages of development will seek to improve visual results and duration of therapeutic action by inhibiting the effects of VEGF-A via other mechanisms.

VEGF-Trap

VEGF-Trap is the first anti-VEGF agent in a class of drugs known as fusion proteins. It is a composite soluble protein that contains genetically engineered DNA portions of the extracellular principal binding domains of VEGF receptors 1 and 2 (VEGFR1 and VEGFR2) and the Fc portion of the human IgG molecule (human IgG1) (180). It binds tightly to all VEGF-A isoforms and both Placental Growth Factor isoforms (PlGF 1 and PlGF 2), and it is this high affinity that allows it to be effective at much lower concentrations than ranibizumab, bevacizumab, or pegaptanib sodium. Because it has the IgG1 portion of the protein and because it is a smaller molecule than the full antibody, VEGF-Trap has a long circulating half-life and presence in the ocular tissues. It would thus be expected to have a longer duration of action. It is currently being evaluated in phase II trials. The phase I trial evaluated the effects of a single intravitreal injection of VEGF-Trap (0.05 mg, 0.15 mg, 0.5 mg, 1.0 mg, 2.0 mg, 4.0 mg) in 21 eyes followed for 6 weeks. Stable or improved vision was seen in 95% of eyes, and the mean best corrected vision after treatment increased by 4.8 letters at 6 weeks for all doses tested. In eyes receiving 2 or 4 mg doses, vision improved by a mean of 13.5 letters, and mean OCT measured retinal thickness decreased by 134 microns. No systemic or significant ocular adverse events were reported (181).

RNA interference (RNAi) or "gene silencing"

Nearly a decade ago, researchers learned that if small double-stranded RNA strands were injected into a cell, they hybridized with endogenous RNA–opening up the possibility that gene expression could be manipulated (182). These segments of RNA were termed small interfering RNAs (siRNAs) (97–99), base pair fragments of double-stranded RNA enzymatically broken down by an RNAase III nuclease. To manipulate gene expression, siRNAs are delivered through the cellular membrane inside the capsid of an adenovirus (183) or retrovirus (184) and then integrated into a cleavage catalyst RNA-induced silencing complex (RISC) to then target and ultimately "silence" specific native mRNA.

Bevasiranib sodium (formerly Cand 5®), developed by Acuity Pharmaceuticals, is the first siRNA molecule tested in the eye. It is intravitreally injected to "silence" the translation of VEGF, and has the potential to more completely eliminate the action of VEGF than agents that act only on previously produced, existing extracellular VEGF. Such complete blockage of the new production of VEGF may be more efficacious in stopping CNV activity. A single bevasiranib molecule can eliminate thousands of VEGF proteins, have a longer duration of action that reduces the frequency of intravitreal injections, and act synergistically with VEGF blockers to thus stop the effect of both new VEGF production and existing VEGF molecules. It is currently being evaluated in phase II clinical trials, after its acceptable phase I safety profile was demonstrated following intravitreal injections of up to 3 mg per eye given at 6-week intervals. Only mild ocular adverse events were reported, and importantly, no systemic exposure to the drug was detected.

The Acuity Cand 5 Anti-VEGF RNAi Evaluation or C.A.R.E. Trial was a phase II safety and efficacy study, the results of which were presented at the 24th Annual Meeting of the American Society of Retina Specialists in Cannes, France in September 2006. This randomized, double-masked, nonplacebo controlled trial was done at 28 sites and evaluated the efficacy of bevasiranib in 129 eyes with either classic or minimally classic CNV, including those that had failed prior treatment. The drug was well tolerated at all doses; no significant increase in ocular or systemic adverse events was noted. Pharmacokinetic studies confirmed that there was no systemic exposure to the drug. Though there was no placebo arm in this study, visual acuity responses in treated eyes were felt to be better than those seen without treatment in the placebo arms of other trials. There was an overall mean loss of vision in the study eyes in the first few months but then there was visual stabilization. This early decrease was attributed to the unblocked effect of existing VEGF molecules, the action of which would not be inhibited by the drug. After visual stabilization, more than one-third of patients exhibited visual improvement, particularly those that received higher doses. Most patients that were in the trial for 6 months did not require rescue therapy with an FDA-approved mode of therapy (185).

Another siRNA molecule in development, Sirna-027 from SiRNA Therapeutics, targets VEGFR1 and has been shown to be well tolerated in a phase I trial and lead to stabilization of vision in 96% of eyes, improvement of 3 lines of vision in 23% of eyes, and a generally reduced mean foveal thickness by OCT at 8 weeks after a single injection (186,187).

Other Angiogenesis Inhibitors

Squalamine lactate is a naturally occurring aminosterol derived from the dogfish shark liver. It inhibits multiple aspects of angiogenesis including activation of growth factors (e.g., VEGF), integrin expression, and cytoskeletal formation. Its action at the intracellular level of the endothelial cells that form CNV causes apoptosis and regression of the neovascular complex. It has been under development as Evizon® for intravenous administration by Genaera Corp., being evaluated for safety and efficacy most recently in several phase II trials. Results to date have demonstrated that systemic intravenous administration of 10 mg and 40 mg doses of squalamine given once a week for 4 weeks led to stable or improved vision in 90% to 100% of eyes and visual improvement of ≥3 lines at the 4-month completion of the study in a significant number of patients. No significant adverse events were reported. A phase III, multicenter, randomized, controlled trial was planned. However, the phase II trials were unable to meet their enrollment goals because of the availability and rapid acceptance of ranibizumab and bevacizumab, and preliminary impressions from investigators suggested that squalamine lactate was not likely to produce enough consistent visual improvement to compete with existing approved drugs. Thus, in early 2007, Genaera Corp. terminated its development of this drug for the treatment of AMD (188).

Pigment-epithelial derived growth factor agents

Pigment-epithelial derived growth factor (PEDF), produced by the pigmented cells of the eye, inhibits endothelial cell migration and angiogenesis, and has neuroprotective effects (189). Retinal cell PEDF is an important part of the normal process of angiogenesis, the production of which correlates with tissue oxygen levels. Hypoxia causes a reduction of PEDF but an increase in VEGF levels. PEDF administered intravitreally in a mouse model of ischemic retinopathy inhibited retinal neovascularization by causing cellular apoptosis (190). Intravitreal and subretinal injection of a PEDF adenoviral vector reduced laser-induced CNV in a mouse CNV model (191). AdPEDF is a gene delivery method being developed by GenVec, Inc., where a replication-deficient adenovirus vector delivers a gene into a cell to produce PEDF and then treat CNV. A phase I trial of 28 eyes with CNV has been initiated. Acceptable safety results and positive visual and anatomic responses have been demonstrated in these eyes that have been followed for 1 year. Preparation is underway for an impending phase II trial (190,192,193).

Kinase inhibitors

Kinase inhibitors interrupt the catalysis of the phosphorylation process required to activate the VEGF receptor, thereby blocking the VEGF-induced activation of endothelial cells that is needed for neovascularization (194,195). Numerous pharmaceutical manufacturers are in the early stages of investigating tyrosine kinase inhibitors, protein kinase C inhibitors, c-Raf kinase inhibitors, and others as potential antiangiogenic agents for AMD.

Vascular disrupting agents

A new class of agents called vascular disrupting agents (VDAs) is being developed for the treatment of diseases marked by abnormal angiogenesis such as cancer and AMD. VDAs attack blood vessels by altering the shape of newly formed endothelial cells from flat to round, which thereby reduces blood flow through the vessel lumen. They do not affect mature endothelial cells or normal tissue. They have been shown to disrupt vascular endothelial-cadherin—a protein found at the endothelial cell junction that is important in endothelial cell survival, migration, and proliferation. Combretastatin A 4 phosphate (CA4P) by Oxigene® is one drug in this class that has been shown to reduce blood flow to tumors. It is currently in phase II clinical trials for the treatment of a number of different types of cancer. The mechanism by which CA4P exerts its antiangiogenic activity in cancer therapy may allow for a similar role in the treatment of neovascular AMD (196,197).

Other novel approaches to neovascular AMD

A possible alternative to intravitreal or intravenous therapy for neovascular AMD is being evaluated by Athenagen, who have developed ATG003, a topical anti-angiogenic eye drop for AMD. It is a proprietary formulation of mecamylamine that inhibits endothelial nicotinic acetylcholine receptors, decreases angiogenesis, and lowers vascular permeability. It is felt to have excellent retinal and choroidal penetration while not significantly entering the systemic circulation. It has shown efficacy in animal models of neovascularization and has recently been evaluated in a dose-escalating phase I trial. Eighty patients were treated twice daily for 14 days. No significant ocular toxicity was noted, and only minimal amounts of drug were found in the systemic circulation. A 330 patient placebo-controlled, double-masked, randomized, dose-ranging phase II trial will begin recruiting in the next few months.

There are drugs in development to target newly described genes that are involved in abnormal angiogenesis. Also, recombinant technology is being applied to the development of anti-VEGF medication with the goal of manufacturing low cost alternative drugs to those currently on the market.

Treatment of Significant Vision Loss From Non-Neovascular AMD

The presence of large drusen is known to be a significant risk factor for the development of CNV, and since resorption of drusen has been noted following focal macular laser, a prospective randomized clinical trial was done to investigate the effects of subthreshold macular laser on eyes with high-risk drusen. Surprisingly, the unilateral arm of the Prophylactic Treatment of AMD Multicenter Trial (PTAMD) showed that at 36 months, laser treatment delivered in a predetermined subthreshold array *increased* the risk of developing CNV, while the bilateral arm demonstrated no such increased neovascular development. No significant visual acuity benefit was gained in either arm of the trial, and thus such therapy for dry high-risk AMD is not currently being pursued (198,199).

Rheophoresis is also being investigated for high-risk non-neovascular AMD. This is a form of therapeutic plasmapharesis that uses two in-line hollow-fiber membrane filters to remove circulating high molecular weight plasma macromolecules that may obstruct choroidal microcirculation. The first filter separates the red and white blood cells from plasma. The plasma is then passed through the second filter where molecules such as alpha-2 macroglobulin, von Willebrand factor, fibrinogen, immune complexes, lipoprotein A, and LDL cholesterol are removed. Small numbers of patients evaluated in early trials have shown some visual improvement with such treatment, although a pivotal prospective, randomized, double-masked, sham-controlled trial, RHEO-AMD, is scheduled to begin recruiting in 2007. It will take place at up to 25 sites where patients will receive either 8 RHEO treatments or eight sham procedures over 10 weeks. As of this writing, no conclusive evidence exists to support the use of rheophoresis for AMD, although the larger phase III trial will expand the evaluation of its efficacy.

The lipid-lowering agents known as statins are being evaluated for their potential to slow or prevent AMD progression because of their antioxidant, anti-inflammatory, anti-angiogenic, and lipid-lowering activity, and because of their potential neuroprotective effects on the photoreceptors.

Other anti-inflammatory agents and even antibiotics are being looked at as potential treatments for advanced AMD.

An innovative surgical device to treat central vision loss from AMD was developed by Isaac Lipshitz, M.D. in the form of the implantable miniature telescope (IMT), currently manufactured by Visioncare Ophthalmic Technologies. Presently, patients with bilateral central disciform scarring or geographic atrophy of the RPE have few treatment options to improve vision. The IMT, a prosthetic telescopic implant, was developed to offer a permanent optical solution for these patients by improving vision by reducing the size of the scotoma relative to objects in the central visual field. It is implanted in place of the crystalline lens during cataract extraction and held in place with haptics. It enlarges images 2.2 or 3 times, depending on the device used, and aims to place images of objects in the central visual field off damaged macular tissue and onto healthier adjacent retina. It is theoretically beneficial when placed in one eye to aid with central vision, while the unimplanted eye provides better peripheral vision. Visual rehabilitation is then done to help patients maximize their visual potential. A prospective, multicenter trial evaluated 217 patients that received the IMT in one eye at 28 sites. At 1 year after IMT implantation, 67% of patients had ≤3 lines of visual improvement vs. 13% of fellow eye controls; 25% achieved ≥5 lines visual improvement vs. 2% of fellow eyes; and 1.6% of patients had a loss of ≥3 lines vs. 3.1% of fellow eyes. Although these results were impressive for a group of patients with heretofore no treatment options, safety concerns prompted the U.S. FDA Ophthalmic Devices Advisory Panel to vote against approval of the IMT because mean corneal endothelial cell counts decreased by more than 25% at 1 year after implantation—20% within the first 3 months (200). A better understanding of the nature of the endothelial cell loss and a subsequent plan to remedy this problem will be required before the IMT can be approved by the FDA. The manufacturer and investigators of the IMT plan continued effort in this direction.

FAILED TREATMENTS FOR NEOVASCULAR AMD

There are several notable treatment approaches that demonstrated initial promise as therapy for CNV but were ultimately shown to not be beneficial in the management of AMD-related vision loss.

Radiation therapy

Considered as a possible treatment for AMD because it rapidly inhibits dividing cells, radiation therapy has been evaluated as a treatment for CNV for over a decade. Radiation has been delivered to the eye by several methods including external beam photon radiation, brachytherapy (sutured external radioactive plaque), and proton beam irradiation (201–203). Although early studies indicated that there may be some benefit to radiation therapy, more recent studies cast doubt on its efficacy. Several small series, both randomized and non-randomized, have shown some success at reducing vision loss (204–209), particularly in eyes with classic CNV, but other recent trials have shown no effect (210–213). Prospective controlled trials have been done. The Radiation Therapy for Age-Related Macular Degeneration Study Group was unable to show a significant treatment benefit with several fractions of low ionizing radiation, nor was Marcus et al (210,215). Two smaller controlled trials using fewer high radiation fractions showed a significant improvement of vision, which prompted the initiation of the ARMD Radiotherapy Trial (ARM-DRT) (216,217). At one year in this study, vision, loss was equal in eyes treated with radiation and control eyes (218).

Transpupillary Thermotherapy (TTT)

TTT is a procedure in which diode laser energy (810 nm) is used to slowly heat the choroid, RPE, and CNV complex to occlude the neovascularization with a single large laser spot while also avoiding thermal damage to the surrounding neurosensory retina and adjacent cells.

Its precise mechanism of action is not known, although it is suspected that it alters choroidal blood flow with its energy spot of largely unknown intensity (219–221). Initial series suggested that TTT was beneficial in the treatment of occult CNV. Reichel et al reported that 94% of eyes treated with TTT had decreased exudation while no eyes suffered adverse effects (222). Thach et al demonstrated that TTT treatment resulted in better outcomes than seen with the natural history of occult CNV (223). In the VIP trial, eyes with occult CNV that received TTT had outcomes equivalent to those receiving PDT at 6 and 12 months (224). The Transpupillary Thermotherapy of Occult Choroidal Neovascular Membranes in Patients with Age-Related Macular Degeneration Trial (TTT4CNV) was a large-scale prospective, randomized, placebo-controlled trial that enrolled 303 patients from 22 sites. It compared TTT vs. sham treatment in eyes with occult subfoveal CNV and moderate vision loss (20/50 to 20/200). Overall, no statistically significant difference was noted between the two groups, although subgroup analysis of eyes with pretreatment vision ≤20/100 showed that TTT offered improved visual acuity at 18 months (225,226). A recent trial showed similar visual improvement and stabilization with TTT in occult CNV. Improved vision was noted in 14% of eyes and stabilization was achieved in 56% at 24 months. Over longer periods of follow-up, increased vision loss was noted (227).

Given the lack of significant visual and anatomic success with TTT, particularly in the setting where the endpoint of treatment (a largely invisible laser spot) is nebulous, and given the development of more obviously successful therapies such as PDT and later anti-VEGF therapy, most retinal physicians have come to abandon TTT for CNV.

Anecortave Acetate

Anecortave acetate, manufactured by Alcon, Inc. as Retaane®, is a novel angiostatic cortisene—a new type of steroid with minimal glucocorticoid and mineralocorticoid activity. It was thought to have potential benefit in the treatment of CNV because of its ability to inhibit extracellular matrix proteolysis and was initially shown to be effective in animal models of neovascularization (228–230). A phase II/III study of 128 eyes with classic subfoveal CNV showed that a 15 mg dose, delivered juxtasclerally with a specially designed cannula, resulted in visual improvement, visual stabilization, and prevention of vision loss that was superior to placebo controls. A phase III noninferiority trial evaluated anecortave acetate injected every 3 months vs. PDT. At 12 months, no difference in the loss of ≤3 lines of vision was seen between the two treatments. The trial did not meet the endpoint of noninferiority, but the FDA gave Alcon, Inc. an approvable letter suggesting that further study was needed to bring the drug to market. It is currently not being developed for the treatment of active CNV, although it is under investigation for the prevention of neovascular AMD (231,232).

PREVENTION OF AMD

Though dramatic improvements in the treatment of neovascular AMD have been achieved in the past two decades—most strikingly in the past few years—the "holy grail" in the management of AMD is prevention.

The Age-Related Eye Disease Study (AREDS)

The first and most significant foray into the area of AMD prevention was an investigation of the relationship between vitamin supplementation and the natural history of AMD. AREDS was a landmark study sponsored by the National Eye Institute to determine possible effects of high-dose antioxidant vitamins and zinc on AMD progression and cataract development. It also sought to provide extensive prospective controlled data on the natural history of untreated AMD. Roughly 4,700 patients between ages 55 and 80 years with AMD characteristics were enrolled. They were classified into one of four groups based on their clinical characteristics and risk for progression (see Diagnosis, pages 19–20). A total of 3,640 patients were divided into 4 groups of approximately 900 patients each and given *placebo, antioxidants, minerals, or antioxidants plus minerals* (Fig. 54). The antioxidant formula contained 500 mg vitamin C, 400 mg (400 IU) vitamin E, and 15 mg beta-carotene (28,640 IU vitamin A). The mineral formula contained 80 mg of zinc oxide and 2 mg of cupric oxide, given to prevent a zinc-induced copper-deficiency anemia. Mean follow-up for the series was 6.3 years. In eyes receiving no supplementation (placebo group), the probability of progressing to advanced AMD (CNV or geographic atrophy involving the foveal center) at 5 years was found to be 1.3% in Group 2 eyes, 18% in Group 3 eyes, and 43% in Group 4 eyes (Fig. 55). Group 2 eyes (extensive small drusen, nonextensive intermediate sized drusen, or only pigmentary abnormalities) had such a low incidence of progression to advanced AMD that the study was unable to shed light on the value of supplementation in these patients or in

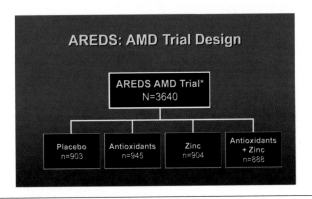

Figure 54. AREDS trial design. From Age-Related Eye Disease Study Research Group. *Arch Opthalmol.* 2001; 199: 1417–1436. Copyright © 2001, American Medical Association. All rights reserved, with permission.

Group 1 patients (those without significant early findings of AMD). Supplementation did not prevent progression from Group 2 to Groups 3 or 4, and therefore Group 1 and 2 eyes were excluded from further analysis. In Groups 3 and 4 eyes that received supplementation, the likelihood of progression to advanced AMD at 5 years was 23% for those taking antioxidants, 22% for those taking minerals only, and 20% for those taking antioxidants plus minerals—compared with 28% for those receiving placebo (Fig. 56). The differences between the rates of progression in the antioxidant plus mineral combination eyes, and minerals only eyes, and those of placebo eyes were statistically significant. The reduction in the risk of developing advanced AMD was 25% for those taking the antioxidant plus minerals, 21% for those taking

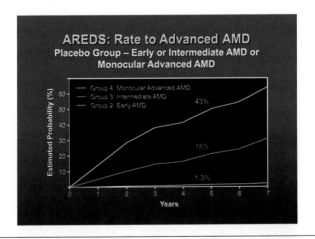

Figure 55. AREDS Results: Probability of progression to advanced AMD, by severity of pre-existing AMD. From Age-Related Eye Disease Study Research Group. *Arch Opthalmol.* 2001; 199: 1417–1436. Copyright © 2001, American Medical Association. All rights reserved, with permission.

minerals alone, and 17% for those taking antioxidants alone (Fig. 57). Visual acuity loss ≥3 lines at 5 years was seen in 23% of those taking the combination of antioxidants and minerals, 25% of those taking minerals alone, 26% of those receiving antioxidants alone, and 29% of those taking placebo (Fig. 58). The difference between placebo and those taking the combination was statistically significant (88,233).

A useful analysis of the AREDS data has led to the development of the AREDS Clinical Severity Scale, which uses simple clinical features to determine disease significance and the relative risk of a vision-threatening event (Tab. 1).

This easy-to-use score allows physicians to accurately and quickly assess patient risk for severe vision-threatening events and direct the level of follow-up based on expected courses of progression.

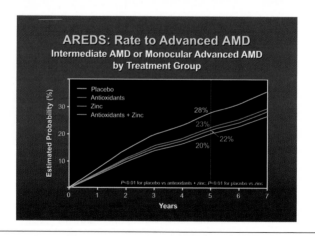

Figure 56. AREDS Results: Probability of progression to advanced AMD, by category of supplement taken. From Age-Related Eye Disease Study Research Group. *Arch Opthalmol.* 2001; 199: 1417–1436. Copyright © 2001, American Medical Association. All rights reserved, with permission.

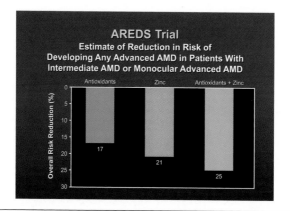

Figure 57. AREDS Results: Reduction in risk of developing advanced AMD, by category of supplement taken. From Age-Related Eye Disease Study Research Group. *Arch Opthalmol.* 2001; 199: 1417–1436.

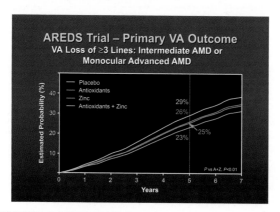

Figure 58. AREDS Results: Probability of VA loss of ≥3 lines, by category of supplement taken. From Age-Related Eye Disease Study Research Group. *Arch Opthalmol.* 2001; 199: 1417–1436. Copyright © 2001, American Medical Association. All rights reserved, with permission.

Table 1	AREDS clinical severity scale (9)

Key value calculated:

<u>Patient severity score</u> = sum or risk factors present in both eyes (0 to 4).

<u>Clinical features:</u>	1) Large drusen – diameter >125 μ (approximately equal to width of a vein at the disc)
	2) Pigmentary changes: hyper- or hypopigmentation
<u>Scoring</u>:	1) Above features count as 1
	2) Advanced AMD counts as 2
	3) If both eyes have extensive intermediate drusen, score = $\frac{1}{2}$ for each eye
	4) Both eyes are scored and the values added to achieve the overall patient severity score

5-Year Risks:	By Patient Severity Score				
Score	0	1	2	3	4
% Risk	0.5	3	12	25	50

AREDS had excellent follow-up and adherence to the assignment of supplements. Few adverse effects were described. Slightly more genitourinary problems were noted in the zinc-only group, and more skin hypersensitivity was seen in the antioxidant group.

In summary, recommendations from this very important study include: (a) Patients with extensive intermediate-sized drusen, at least one large druse, noncentral geographic atrophy of the RPE, monocular advanced AMD, or vision loss from AMD in one eye—and who are non-smokers—will benefit from taking antioxidants plus zinc and copper to reduce the likelihood of disease progression and loss of vision; (b) Patients with early stage AMD have a low enough risk of progression to advanced disease that they do not receive enough benefit to need supplementation until they progress to a more intermediate stage of AMD.

Another major study looking at vitamin supplementation in AMD patients, The Rotterdam Study, found that high dietary intake of antioxidants such as those in the AREDS formulation (vitamin C, vitamin E, beta-carotene, and zinc) reduced the risk of AMD in the elderly by 35%. The amount of nutrients taken in this population was much less than the doses taken in the AREDS trial, but yet the apparent protective effects of these nutrients were still seen (234).

It is estimated that roughly 300,000 patients could avoid advanced AMD during a 5-year period if all eligible AMD patients followed AREDS' recommendations. It is important to note that none of the supplements can restore lost vision or alter the course of cataract progression (88).

Questions exist surrounding the study recommendations. It is not known if there are any deleterious effects of taking such supplementation for longer than 7 years, if using different doses of these components or changes to the formulation would alter the benefit seen in the trial, or if patients with early AMD would not get some benefit from supplementation if taken for a longer period of time.

A more recent evaluation of the AREDS data provided interesting correlations between supplementation and morbidity and mortality rates. Those taking AREDS recommended vitamin and mineral supplementation had a 14% reduction in mortality compared with placebo controls. Patients with advanced AMD were 1.4 times more likely to die than those with few or no drusen and had a higher rate of cardiovascular death in particular. Patients with vision <20/40, nuclear cataracts, or cataract extraction had higher all-cause and cancer mortality rates. Those taking zinc had lower mortality than those not taking zinc (233,235).

A number of potentially modifiable lifestyle choices, behaviors, and physical characteristics have been shown to be risk factors for

AMD. Cigarette smoking is a well-demonstrated risk factor for AMD development. Current smokers have been shown to be at higher risk for incident AMD than past smokers and those that have never smoked (236). A recent paper published by Seddon et al describes the results of an observational analysis of a unique cohort of elderly male twins from the U.S. Twin Study of Age-Related Macular Degeneration. A total of 222 eyes with intermediate or advanced AMD and 459 eyes with early or no disease were followed. Current smokers were found to have an increased AMD risk of 1.9 times, and past smokers of 1.7 times, compared with nonsmokers (237). This may occur because of the negative effect of smoking on antioxidant metabolism and choroidal blood flow (238). There are other modifiable lifestyle behaviors that may affect AMD development and progression. Higher waist circumference has been associated with twice the risk of advanced AMD ($P=0.02$) (239). Specific dietary factors have also been associated with increased AMD. Total fat consumption (relative risk = 2.90, 95% C.I.) has been strongly correlated with a higher risk of developing advanced AMD. Higher intake of both animal fat (relative risk = 2.29, 95% C.I.) and vegetable fat (relative risk = 3.82, 95% C.I.) has been correlated with increased AMD progression, as has consumption of saturated, monounsaturated, polyunsaturated, and transunsaturated fats. Increased consumption of baked goods doubled the risk of AMD progression whereas consumption of fish and nuts was protective against progression, (240). Cho et al reported that high linoleic acid intake was associated with a 49% increased risk of AMD, whereas high DHA (docosahexaenoic acid) intake (an omega-3 fatty acid found in fish or supplements) was associated with a 30% reduction of AMD risk (241). In the Seddon trial that reported results from the Twins Study, it was reported that consumption of fish, particularly two or more servings per week, and increased omega-3 fatty acid dietary intake was associated with decreased AMD development (237).

Micronutrients such as the plant carotenoid pigments lutein and zeaxanthin, found in green leafy vegetables, corn, egg yolks, squash, peas, and others, may be modifiable dietary or supplemental factors that could potentially impact AMD. Data from AREDS demonstrated that high levels of lutein and zeaxanthin were protective against AMD. Those with intermediate or advanced AMD (AREDS categories 3 and 4) with the highest dietary intake of both pigments had a decreased risk of developing neovascular AMD and geographic RPE atrophy. Those with diets high in omega-3 fatty acids DHA and EPA (eicosapentaenoic acid) had reduced risk of developing neovascular AMD and geographic RPE atrophy (242). Results from the recently reported CAREDS trial (Carotenoids in Age-Related Eye Disease Study) support previous assertions about these pigments. Healthy women less than 75 years old with a higher dietary intake of lutein and zeaxanthin (3 or more mg/day) had a 43% reduced risk for the development of intermediate or advanced AMD compared with controls (dietary intake $\leq^3/_4$ mg/day) (243).

With the goal of refining and expanding upon the findings of the original AREDS, a new NIH-sponsored national prospective randomized trial, AREDS 2, is being initiated. Specifically, the addition of the carotenoid pigments and omega-3 fatty acids to the known vitamin and mineral supplement will be evaluated. The effect of supplementation of 10 mg lutein, 2 mg zeaxanthin, 1 g DHA/EPA, the combination of all the above, and placebo on moderate vision loss, progression of AMD along the AREDS AMD scale, cataract surgery, and cognitive function will be evaluated in 4,000 patients over the next several years.

A second AREDS 2 randomization will evaluate the effects of manipulating the carotene and low dose zinc levels in the supplements.

Exercise may be protective against AMD. Researchers have demonstrated that physical activity (vigorous activity 3 times per week) is associated with a 25% reduced risk of AMD progression compared with those who do not regularly exercise (239). Researchers reported 15-year data from the Beaver Dam Eye Study of 3,874 participants living in Beaver Dam, Wisconsin, and showed that those who participated in regular activity 3 times per week had a 70% risk reduction for the development of neovascular AMD than those without an active lifestyle (no regular activity with sweating 3 or more times per week) after multivariate analysis controlled for age, gender, arthritis, blood pressure, body mass index, smoking, and education. An increase in the number of blocks walked per day correlated with a decreased risk of neovascular AMD. Increased walking of more than 12 blocks per day reduced the incidence of neovascular AMD by 30%. Activity was not related to the incidence of early AMD or geographic RPE atrophy (244).

Anecortave Acetate

The angiostatic cortisene anecortave acetate is being evaluated as a potential pharmacologic prophylactic for neovascular AMD in the Alcon, Inc. supported Anecortave Acetate Risk Reduction Trial (AART). Its safety and efficacy have been well described in the phase III trial for neovascular AMD treatment. In this trial, it is administered into a posterior juxtascleral location presumably near the macula in high-risk eyes with at least five drusen and focal hyperpigmentation of patients with a fellow eye that has neovascular AMD. The goal of the trial is to determine if the drug can entirely prevent the development of CNV in these high-risk eyes. This is an ongoing trial, the results of which will not be known for several years.

Patient Care Issues

George A. Williams

The visual complications of age-related macular degeneration are frustrating and sometimes devastating to afflicted patients. The recent publicity concerning the substantial treatment benefits of ranibizumab and bevacizumab has generated great hope and sometimes unrealistic expectations among patients. Patients now often present with the expectation of significant visual improvement. Patients with neovascular AMD presenting to ophthalmologists require a detailed discussion of the natural history of the disease, the potential visual outcomes and risks of treatment, and the extent of the treatment burden. The overall challenge is to extrapolate the results of clinical trials or clinical reports to an individual patient. This requires that the ophthalmologist explain that clinical trial results are only applicable to patients presenting with similar disease to those individuals studied in the trials. For example, patients with long-term, severe visual loss and end-stage neovascular scars cannot be expected to respond as well, if at all, as individuals with more recent disease. Even for patients with earlier disease, it is important to stress that visual loss is still possible (about 30% chance) and that significant visual improvement (≥3 lines) occurs in a minority (30% to 40%) of patients. The ophthalmologist must also ascertain that the patient understands and is able and willing to comply with the treatment plan. For anti-VEGF therapy, this involves multiple injections, imaging studies, and office visits at approximately monthly intervals for 1 to 2 years. The logistical issues of travel and time for the patient and often their family must be explained. Patients often assume that because they have heard that ranibizumab or other therapy restored reading or driving in some individuals, that they will have a similar benefit. However, even a 3-line improvement in someone starting with ≤20/200 vision in their better eye is unlikely to restore such function. Even sophisticated patients struggle to understand concepts such as less than three-line loss or more than three-line gain. It is helpful to explain these changes in terms of being able to see objects twice as big (3-line loss) or half the size (3-line gain) of those seen prior to starting treatment.

One useful technique to help patients understand their treatment chances is the number needed to treat (NNT) (245). NNT is an estimate of the number of patients who need to be treated for one additional patient to benefit from a specific outcome. The ideal NNT is one meaning that every patient treated would have the desired benefit. For ranibizumab, the NNT to treat for a 3-line improvement at one year is 2.9 in the ANCHOR study and 3.5 in the MARINA study. When compared with NNT for a similar response with pegaptanib in the VISION study, 25, the treatment benefit becomes readily apparent.

Despite the best available treatment, some patients will have a suboptimal response and become discouraged and even depressed. Based on the Hospital Anxiety and Depression Scale, up to one quarter of patients with newly diagnosed CNV have measurable anxiety and depression (246). As expected, median anxiety and depression scores are worse for patients with bilateral disease (247). In a recent study of 13,900 people aged 75 years and older, visually impaired people had a higher prevalence of depression as measured by the Geriatric

Depression Scale compared with people with good vision (13.5% vs. 4.6%). Of patients with best bilateral visual acuity of less than 20/60 due to AMD, 15.1% were depressed (248). Patients who fail to respond to treatment can be expected to do even worse. An effective low vision services program involving visual aides, preferential visual locus training, and support groups can be invaluable for many patients (249, 250). Psychiatric evaluation is appropriate for patients with clinically significant depression.

Quality of Life

George A. Williams

Quality of life (QOL) measurements are becoming increasingly important in the evaluation and management of a host of chronic disease states including age-related macular degeneration. QOL describes the ability of individuals to participate in common activities of daily living such as driving, reading, and recognizing faces. Although QOL of life measurements are patient derived and, therefore, subjective, they can provide valuable information on the personal impact of a disease state and its treatment (251).

In AMD, QOL has been measured with the National Eye Institute Visual Function Questionnaire (NEI-VFQ) (252). The NEI-VFQ is a validated instrument that assesses general health, visual health, pain, and near and distance visual activities. The NEI-VFQ also measures how visual disability affects mental health, role difficulties, social functioning and dependency, driving, and color and peripheral vision. Scores range from 0–100 (worse to best level of function). A 10-point change is the equivalent of a 3-line change in vision. In AMD, patients with bilateral visual loss score worse than those with monocular loss even after correcting for visual acuity. In patients with bilateral severe AMD, the mean QOL scores using the NEI-VFQ for quality of vision and vision specific subscales are significantly worse than for patients with AMD of varying severity or persons without eye disease (253). Furthermore, QOL decreases significantly in persons with declining visual acuity (254).

In persons with AMD, the inability to drive or fear of not being able to drive is a critical issue. There is a direct correlation between higher severity of AMD and poorer scores on the driving activities subscale of the Activities of Daily vision Scale, a 21 item questionnaire about vision activities such as driving. The loss of driving ability can decrease the ability to care for oneself or others (255). This loss of independence can be devastating both emotionally and financially and increases the risk of social isolation. Not surprising, AMD may lead to depression and anxiety. In the Submacular Surgery Trials, there was a 13% incidence of anxiety and 12% incidence of depression as measured by the Hospital Anxiety and Depression Scale (247). In another study, patients with severe bilateral AMD scored significantly lower in the social and mental health domains of NEI-VFQ-25 than patients with AMD of varying severity and persons without ocular disease (143,144). Visual loss from age-related macular degeneration may also cause cognitive impairment. In the AREDS, persons with vision worse than 20/40 in both eyes were more likely to be cognitively impaired (OR, 2.88; 95% CI, 1.75–4.76) compared with persons with better visual acuity (256). Another study demonstrated cognitive impairment in 18% of persons with late AMD compared with 2.6% of persons without AMD (257).

Importantly, the perception of people with AMD about the impact of their visual loss upon their quality of life is different from that of nonafflicted people, nonophthalmologist clinicians, and even ophthalmologists who treat people with AMD as measured by a time tradeoff utility analysis (258). In a time tradeoff utility analysis, a person is asked how long he or she expects to live. The person is then asked what is the maximum amount of that remaining life span he or she is willing to trade for a return to normal health during the years that remain. The utility value associated with disease is then calculated by subtracting the proportion of time traded from 1.00. For example, if a patient with AMD who expects to live 10 years is willing to trade 3 of those years for a return to normal vision, the utility value is 0.70 (1.00–0.30). Utility analysis values obtained from large populations are reproducible. Ophthalmic utility values best correlate with visual acuity in the better-seeing eye, rather than the cause of visual loss. The values range from 1.00 for 20/20 vision in each eye permanently to 0.54 for 20/400 and 0.26 for no light perception. In this analysis, a person who loses vision from 20/20 (utility value 1.0) to 20/400 (utility value 0.54) in their better-seeing eye experience a 46% decrease in quality of life. Utility values associated with visual loss from AMD correlate with the severity of visual loss and are comparable with the utility value of other severe, chronic diseases. For moderate AMD (20/50 to 20/100), the mean utility value of 0.68 is similar to that following a moderate stroke. For severe AMD (20/200 or worse), the mean utility value of 0.47 is similar to the QOL associated with total renal failure on home dialysis. Very severe AMD (20/800 or worse) is associated with a QOL comparable with a severe stroke or advanced prostate cancer with uncontrolled pain (259).

The difference in the perception of how neovascular AMD affects QOL is dramatic between patients and ophthalmologists who treat AMD. Even for mild AMD (visual acuity 20/20 to 20/40) the patient estimated decrease in the remaining QOL was 17% compared with 2% for ophthalmologists. For moderate visual loss (visual acuity of 20/50 to 20/100) the difference was a decrement of 32% vs. 11%. For severe AMD (visual acuity 20/200 or worse) the difference was 53% vs. 27%, and for visual acuity of 20/800 or less the difference was 60% vs. 33%. This means the average ophthalmologist when asked to assess the quality of life associated with very severe AMD was willing to trade approximately 3.3 of every remaining 10 years for a return to normal vision compared with the average afflicted patient with very severe AMD who was willing to trade 6.1 of every remaining year for the same result (258, 259). These data clearly warn ophthalmologists not to underestimate the devastating impact of neovascular AMD on their patients' quality of life.

These utility values can also be used to measure the improvement in QOL associated with a treatment. For example, an improvement from 20/400 (utility value = 0.54) to 20/40 (utility value = 0.80) results in 0.26 gain in utility value and 48% (0.26/0.54) gain in QOL. Once the utility value gain of a treatment is established, the total value can be determined in quality-adjusted-life-years (QALY). The formula for QALY is utility value x number of years. For AMD, the formula to measure the total value gained from a treatment is:

(utility value gain from treatment) × (duration of treatment benefit in years)

Once the total value in QALY is known, cost utility of treatments can be calculated. This requires modeling, which considers the costs of the treatment such as drug costs and the effects of treatment-related complications, imaging costs, and practice overhead (260). Also, the frequency of treatment over time is considered. For example, in the clinical trials for PDT, the number of treatments per year decreased from year 1 to year 5. The cost utility analysis generates the cost per QALY, which can then be compared with recognized standards for cost-effectiveness. For neovascular AMD, PDT has been shown to be cost-effective, particularly in persons with relatively good baseline visual acuity (261–264). Cost utility analysis for newer treatments such as ranibizumab are pending. However, because of the increased chance for visual improvement, and therefore increased utility, it is likely that despite the higher costs of ranibizumab, it will prove to be cost-effective as well.

QOL of life indices can also be used to measure and value the impact of therapeutic intervention (265,266). In one study, the relative increase in QOL for PDT ranged from 4.2% to 25.7% (267). In another study, patients treated with PDT were significantly less anxious and more independent outdoors after 1-year of follow-up (268). QOL of life analysis for ranibizumab is ongoing, but preliminary reports also demonstrate QOL improvement in some patients. In the MA-RINA trial, the NEI VFQ 25 measured treatment-related changes in QOL. The mean pretreatment measurement was 60. In patients for whom the treated eye was their better seeing eye, treatment resulted in a nearly 20 point improvement in the near activities subscale compared with controls. For all treated patients, there was a greater than 10-point improvement compared with controls for near activities, distance activities, and vision-specific dependency (269). These improvements signify a substantial improvement in QOL.

QOL studies clearly indicate that even AMD patients with limited visual acuity highly value their remaining vision (270). Ophthalmologists must understand that for many persons preservation of remaining vision is a worthwhile goal. Considering the high value that people ascribe to their vision, ophthalmologists must be careful when recommending unproven or potentially dangerous therapies and should provide patients an evidence-based discussion of the efficacy and safety of therapy whenever possible.

The Economics of AMD

George A. Williams

The economics of AMD can be considered from both a microeconomic and a macroeconomic perspective. The microeconomic perspective involves costs from the individual perspective of the patient and the ophthalmologist. The macroeconomic perspective involves the costs to society and the health care system. Together, these costs pose significant and difficult issues for patients, ophthalmologists, and society.

The economic burden to the patient of treatment for neovascular AMD can be considerable. Although most patients with neovascular AMD have Medicare, patients are responsible for 20% of the cost of evaluation and management services, ocular imaging, intraocular injections, photodynamic laser and physician-administered (Part B) drugs. For ranibizumab, this can total $400 to $500 per month. The need for repeated treatment in many patients multiplies the economic burden. Fortunately, a majority of Americans have supplemental insurance to cover these copayment costs. Additionally, most drug companies have programs to assist financially eligible patients with drug-related copayments. There can also be significant indirect costs associated with neovascular AMD including transportation, parking, time off of work, or even loss of a job. The net result is that treatment of neovascular AMD can create a substantial economic burden for many patients.

For ophthalmologists, treatment of neovascular AMD creates significant economic issues as well. Practice management issues involving increased patient volume and drug costs are considerable. The increased patient volume may require additional office and clinical personnel. The cost of drugs such as ranibizumab distort practice accounting and necessitate detailed following of accounts payable and receivable. Under Medicare regulations, the allowable reimbursement for ranibizumab is the average sales price plus a 6% margin. For the first 6 months of ranibizumab use, the allowable reimbursement was $2,067. However, on January 1, 2007, the reimbursement dropped to $2,036. This was due to the costs of distributing the drug through wholesalers. These costs decrease the average sales price and therefore the allowable reimbursement. The average sales price is recalculated every 6 months, meaning that further changes are possible. Additionally, state and local sales taxes or gross revenue taxes on drug costs or revenue can further decrease the net reimbursement to the ophthalmologist. Medicare pays 80% of the allowable reimbursement for ranibizumab. The ophthalmologist's cost for ranibizumab is $1,950. Thus it is essential that the 20% copayment be collected. Unfortunately, this may be difficult due to vagaries of secondary insurance coverage and patients' inability to pay. Ophthalmologists are then placed in the uncomfortable position of losing hundreds of dollars per treatment. This has the potential to create an adversarial situation that may compromise the physician-patient relationship. It is therefore critical that ophthalmologists explain to their patients the financial implications of treatment.

At the macroeconomic level, neovascular AMD is a disease state with a large and increasing case number and effective but expensive treatments resulting in increased utilization of physician services, imaging, and drugs. It is certain, therefore, that the direct costs of treatment of neovascular AMD will total billions of dollars per year and contribute to the continuing escalation in health care costs. Currently, increasing Part B drug costs and physician services adversely affect the sustainable growth rate, which is used to determine yearly reevaluation of physician reimbursement. At present, substantial reductions in physician reimbursement are predicted for the next several years. How long this situation will continue is uncertain, but legislative solutions are under consideration.

Although the direct costs of treatment for neovascular AMD are large, the indirect costs of untreated AMD with attendant blindness, disability, and lost productivity are even greater. People with visual loss from AMD have a lower employment rate than unaffected people. The employment rate for people afflicted with AMD is 44% for those with mild visual limitation and 31% for those with severe visual limitation due to neovascular AMD and/or geographic atrophy compared with 78% of those unaffected. Additionally, people with advanced AMD earn less money compared with those who have no disabilities. In 1997, the mean wage for a person with no disabilities was $31,182. Comparatively, the mean wage for a person with mild visual loss was 30% less, and for a person with severe visual loss it was 38% less. A detailed analysis of the economic loss to the GDP of the United States from AMD estimated the total loss from neovascular and dry AMD to be $29.8 billion. A study in Canada on the effect of AMD upon the Canadian GDP yielded similar results when adjusted for the population difference (271).

Furthermore, vision loss leads to higher noneye related medical care costs due to depression, injury from falls, skilled nursing facility utilization, and long-term care facility admission. A study examining the association between vision loss and medical care costs in Medicare beneficiaries concluded that persons with vision loss incur significantly higher costs than those with normal vision. Approximately 90% of these costs are noneye related medical costs. This study estimated blindness and vision loss resulted in $2.14 billion in non–eye–related medical costs in 2003 (272). Treatments which can retard or reverse vision loss should reduce these costs. Therefore, any analysis of the costs of treating neovascular AMD must consider not only the direct treatments costs but also the above indirect costs associated with vision loss.

A Final Word

Tarek S. Hassan

In this overview of wet AMD, we have seen that the last several years have been a time of significantly increased understanding of many aspects of this disease. As researchers and clinicians, we now expect to control the vision loss from choroidal neovascularization and possibly reverse it. New treatments have transformed the mood of the waiting room filled with wet AMD patients from the general sadness and resignation of fighting an uphill battle against near-certain vision loss, to the confidence, hope, and expectation of success as we turn the tables on the disease. This fundamental leap forward in our thinking, and that of afflicted patients, represents only the beginning of a new era of pursuit of ever-improving vision, a cure for wet AMD, and, ultimately, the prevention of the potentially devastating effects of any form of AMD. The pace of change is increasingly rapid, and for the first time, the lofty goal of "beating AMD" is beginning to come into view.

References

1. Resnikoff S, Pascolini D, Etya'ale D, et al. Global data on visual impairment in the year 2002. *Bull World Health Organ* 2004;82:844–851.
2. Congdon N, O'Colmain B, Klaver CC, et al. Causes and prevalence of visual impairment among adults in the United States. *Arch Ophthalmol* 2004;122:477–485.
3. Friedman DS, O'Colmain BJ, Munoz B, et al. Prevalence of age-related macular degeneration in the United States. *Arch Ophthalmol* 2004;122:564–572.
4. Desai MPL, Lentzner H, Robinson KH. Trends in vision and hearing among older Americans: Aging trends. Hyattsville, MD: National Center for Health Statistics; 2001.
5. Klein R, Klein BE, Linton KL. Prevalence of age-related maculopathy. The Beaver Dam Eye Study. *Ophthalmology* 1992;99(6):933–943.
6. Rogers CC. Food Review. Economic Research Service, USDA. Sept 2002;25:2–7.
7. Klein R, Klein BE, Tomany SC, et al. Ten-year incidence and progression of age-related maculopathy: The Beaver Dam Eye Study. *Ophthalmology* 2002;109:1767–1779.
8. Davis MD, Gangnon RE, Lee LY, et al. The Age-Related Eye Disease Study severity scale for age-related macular degeneration: AREDS Report No. 17. *Arch Ophthalmol* 2005;123:1484–1498.
9. Ferris FL, Davis MD, Clemons TE, et al. A simplified severity scale for age-related macular degeneration: AREDS Report No. 18. *Arch Ophthalmol* 2005;123:1570–1574.
10. Bressler NM. Early detection and treatment of neovascular age-related macular degeneration. *J Am Board Fam Pract* 2002;15:142–152.
11. Bressler SB, Bressler NM, Fine SL, et al. Natural course of choroidal neovascular membranes within the foveal avascular zone in senile macular degeneration. *Am J Ophthalmol* 1982;93:157–163.
12. Gorin MB. A clinician's view of the molecular genetics of age-related maculopathy. *Arch Ophthalmol* 2007;125(January):21.
13. Ambati J, Ambati BK, Yoo SH, et al. Age-related macular degeneration: Etiology pathogenesis, and therapeutic strategies. *Survey of Ophthalmology* 2003;48(3):257.

14. Hageman GS, Mullins RF, Russell SR, et al. Vitronectin is a constituent of ocular drusen and the vitronectin gene is expressed in human retinal pigmented epithelial cells. *FASEB J* 1999; 13:477–484.
15. Grossniklaus HE, Green WR. Choroidal neovascularization. *Am J Ophthalmol* 2004;137:496.
16. Mullins RF, Russell SR, Anderson DH, et al. Drusen associated with aging and age-related macular degeneration contain proteins common t extracellular deposits associated with atherosclerosis, elastosis, amyloidosis, and dense deposit disease. *FASEB J* 2000;14:835.
17. Sarks JP, Sarks SH, Killingsworth MC. Evolution of soft drusen in age-related macular degeneration. *Eye* 1994;8(Pt 3):269.
18. Winkler B, Boulton ME, Gottsch JD et al. Oxidative damage and age-related macular degeneration. *Mol Vis* 2007;5:32.
19. Hageman GS, Luthert PJ, Victor-Chong NH, et al. An integrated hypothesis that considers drusen as biomarkers of immune-mediated processes at the REP-Bruch's membrane interface in aging and age-related macular degeneration. *Prog Retin Eye Res* 2001; 20(6):705.
20. Complications of Age-Related Macular Degeneration Prevention Trial Research Group. Laser treatment in patients with bilateral large drusen: The complications of age-related macular degeneration prevention trial. *Ophthalmology* 2006;113(11):1974.
21. Friberg TR, Musch DC, Lim JI, et al. Prophylactic treatment of age-related macular degeneration report number 1: 810-nanometer laser to eyes with drusen. Unilaterally eligible patients. *Ophthalmology* 2006;113(4); 622.e1.
22. Yannuzzi L, Negrao S, Lida T, et al. Retinal angiomatous proliferation in age-related macular degeneration. *Retina* 2001;21: 416.
23. Holz FG, Pauleikhoff D, Klein R, et al. Pathogenesis of lesions in late age-related macular disease. *Ophthalmology* 2004;137: 504.
24. Friedman DS, O'Colmain BJ, Munoz B, et al. Eye Diseases Prevalence Research Group. Prevalence of age-related macular degeneration in the United States. *Arch Ophthalmol* 2004;122(4):564.
25. Klein R, Klein BE, Linton KL. Prevalence of age-related maculopathy. The Beaver Dam Eye Study. *Ophthalmology* 1992;99:933.
26. Klein R, Klein BE, Knudtson MD, et al. Fifteen-year cumulative incidence of age-related macular degeneration. *Ophthalmology* 2007;114:253.

27. Wang JJ, Rochtchina E, Lee AJ, et al. Ten-year incidence of progression of age-related maculopathy. *Ophthalmology* 2007;114:92.

28. Varma R, Fraser-Bell S, Tan S, et al. *Prevalence of age-related macular degeneration in Latinos: the Los Angeles Latino Eye Study.* Ophthalmology, 2004; 111:1288.

29. Cruickshanks KJ, Hamman RF, Klein R, et al. The prevalence of age-related maculopathy by geographic region and ethnicity: The Colorado-Wisconsin Study of Age-Related Maculopathy. *Arch Ophthalmol* 1997;115: 242.

30. The Eye Disease Case-Control Study Group. Risk factors for neovascular age-related macular degeneration. *Arch Ophthalmol* 1992;110:1701.

31. Klein R, Klein BE, Tomany SC, et al. Ten-year incidence and progression of age-related maculopathy: The Beaver Dam Eye Study. *Ophthalmology* 2002;109:1767.

32. Klein R, Klein BE, Tomany SC, et al. Ten-year incidence of age-related maculopathy and smoking and drinking: The Beaver Dam Eye Study. *Am J Epidemiol* 2002;156:589–598.

33. Age-related Eye Diseases Study Research Group. Risk factors for the incidence of advanced age-related macular degeneration in the Age-Related Eye Disease Study (AREDS). AREDS Report No. 19. *Ophthalmology* 2005;112(4):533.

34. Mitchell P, Wang JJ, Foran S, et al. Five-year incidence of age-related maculopathy lesions: The Blue Mountains Eye Study. *Ophthalmology* 2002;109:1092.

35. Buch H, Vinding T, la Cour M, et al. Risk factors for age-related maculopathy in a 14-year follow up study: The Copenhagen City Eye Study. *Acta Ophthalmol Scand* 2005;83:409.

36. Bok D. Contributions of genetics to our understanding of inherited monogenic retinal diseases and age-related macular degeneration. *Arch Ophthalmol* 2007;125(2):160.

37. Mitchell P, Wang JJ, Smith W, et al. Smoking and the 5-year incidence of age-related maculopathy: The Blue Mountains Eye Study. *Arch Ophthalmol* 2002;120:357.

38. Thornton J, Edwards R, Mitchell P, et al. Smoking and age-related macular degeneration: A review of association. *Eye* 2005; 19(9):935.

39. DeAngelis MM, Ji F, Kim IK, et al. Cigarette smoking, CFH, APOE, ELOVL4, and risk of neovascular age-related macular degeneration. *Arch Ophthalmol* 2007;125(January):49.

40. Seddon JE, Willett W, Speizer FE, et al. A prospective study of cigarette smoking and age-related macular degeneration in women. *JAMA* 1996;276:1141.

41. Hyman L, Schachat AP, He Q, et al. Age-Related Macular Degeneration Risk Factors Study Group. Hypertension, cardiovascular disease, and age-related macular degeneration. *Arch Ophthalmol* 2000;117:351.

42. van Leeuwen R, Ikram MK, Vingerling JR, et al. Blood pressure, atherosclerosis, and the incidence of age-related maculopathy: The Rotterdam Study. *Invest Ophthalmol Vis Sci* 2003;44:3771.

43. Klein R, Klein BE, Tomany SC, et al. The association of cardiovascular disease with the long-term incidence of age-related maculopathy: The Beaver Dam Eye Study. *Ophthalmology* 2003;110:1273.

44. Klein R, Peto T, Bird AC, et al. Perspective: The epidemiology of age-related macular degeneration. *Am J Ophthalmol* 2004;137:486.

45. Tan JS, Mitchell P, Smith W, et al. Cardiovascular risk factors and the long-term incidence of age-related macular degeneration: The Blue Mountains Eye Study. *Ophthalmology* 2007. Epub ahead of print.

46. Hall NF, Gale CR, Syddall H, et al. Risk of macular degeneration in users of statins: cross sectional study. *Br J Ophthalmol* 2001;323:375.

47. Smeeth L, Cook C, Chakravarthy U, et al. A case control study of age-related macular degeneration and use of statins. *Br J Ophthalmol* 2005;89:1171.

48. Klein R, Klein BE, Tomany SC, et al. Relation of statin use to the 5-year incidence and progression of age-related maculopathy. *Arch Ophthalmol* 2003;121:1151.

49. van Leeuwen R, Tomany SC, Wang JJ, et al. Is medication use associated with the incidence of early age-related maculopathy? Pooled findings from 3 continents. *Ophthalmology* 2004;111:1169.

50. Seddon JE, George S, Rosner B, et al. CFH gene variant, Y402H, and smoking, body mass index, environmental associations with advanced age-related macular degeneration. *Hum Hered* 2006;61(3):157.

51. Seddon JE, Rosner B, Sperduto RD, et al. Dietary fat and risk for advanced age-related macular degeneration. *Arch Ophthalmol* 2001; 119(8):1191.

52. Seddon JE, George S, Rosner B. Cigarette smoking, fish consumption, omega-3 fatty acid intake, and associations with age-related macular degeneration: The US Twin Study of Age-Related Macular Degeneration. *Arch Ophthalmol* 2006; 124(7):995.

53. van Leeuwen R, Boekhoorn S, Vingerling JR, et al. Dietary intake of antioxidants and risk of age-related macular degeneration. *JAMA* 2005;294:3101.

54. Chua B, Flood V, Rochtchina E, et al. Dietary fatty acids and the 5-year incidence of age-related maculopathy. *Arch Ophthalmol* 2006; 127(7): 981.

55. Hodge WG, Schachter HM, Lowcock EC, et al. Evidence for the effect of ω3 fatty acids on progression of age-related macular degeneration: A Systematic Review. *RETINA* 2007;27:216.

56. Pollack A, Burkelman A, Zalish M, et al. The course of age-related macular degeneration following bilateral cataract surgery. *Ophthalmic Surg Lasers* 1998;29:286.

57. Freeman EE, Munoz B, West SK, et al. Is there an association between cataract surgery and age-related macular degeneration? Data from three population-based studies. *Am J Ophthalmol* 2003;135:849.

58. Klein R, Klein BE, Wong TY, et al. The association of cataract and cataract surgery with the long-term incidence of age-related maculopathy: the Beaver Dam Eye Study. *Arch Ophthalmol* 2002;120:1551.

59. Wang JJ, Klein RJ, Smith W, et al. Cataract surgery and the 5-year incidence of late-stage age-related maculopathy: pooled findings from the Beaver Dam and Blue Mountains eye studies. *Ophthalmology* 2003; 110(10):1960.

59b. Martin DF, Gensler G, Klein BE for the AREDS Research Group. The effect of cataract surgery on progression to advanced AMD. *Invet Ophthalmol Vis Sci* 2002;43(e-abstract):1907.

60. Ambrecht AM, Findlay C, Aspinall PA, et al. Do patients with age-related maculopathy and cataract benefit from cataract surgery? *Br J Ophthalmol* 1999;83:253.

61. Cugati S, Mitchell P, Rochtchina E, et al. Cataract surgery and the 10-year incidence of age-related maculopathy: the Blue Mountain Eye Study. *Ophthalmology* 2006;113(11):2020.

62. Shuttleworth GN, Luhishi EA, Harrad RA. Do patients with age-related maculopathy and cataract benefit from cataract surgery? *Br J Ophthalmol* 1998;82(June):611.

63. Klaver CC, Wolfs RC, Assink JJ, et al. Genetic risk of age-related maculopathy. Population-based familial aggregation study. *Arch Ophthalmol* 1998;116:1646.

64. Klein BE, Klein R, Lee KE, et al. Risk of incident age-related eye diseases in people with an affected sibling: the Beaver Dam Eye Study. *Am J Epidemiol* 2001;154:207-211.

65. Seddon JM, Ajani UA, Mitchell BD. Familial aggregation of age-related maculopathy. *Am J Ophthalmol* 1997;123:199–206.

66. Seddon JE, Cote J, Page WF, et al. The US twin study of age-related macular degeneration: Relative roles of genetic and environmental influences. *Arch Ophthalmol* 2005;123(3):321.

67. Edwards AO, Ritter R, III Abel KJ, et al. Complement factor H polymorphism and age-related macular degeneration. *Science* 2005;308:421.

68. Klein RJ, Zeiss C, Chew EY, et al. Complement factor H polymorphism in age-related macular degeneration. *Science* 2005;308:385.

69. Haines JL, Hauser MA, Schmidt S, et al. Complement factor H variant increases the risk of age-related macular degeneration. *Science* 2005;308:419.

70. Jakovsdottir J, Conley YP, Weeks DE, et al. Susceptibility genes for age-related maculopathy on chromosome 10q26. *Am J Hum Genet* 2005;77:389.

71. Shuler RK, Jr Hauser MA, Caldwell J, et al. Neovascular age-related macular degeneration and its association with LOC387715 and complement factor H polymorphism. *Arch Ophthalmol* 2007;125 (January):63.

72. Hageman GS, Anderson DH, Johnson LV, et al. A common haplotype in the complement regulatory gene factor H (HF1/CFH) predisposes individuals to age-related macular degeneration. *PNAS* 2005;102 (20):7227.

73. Schaumberg DA, Hankinson SE, Guo Q, et al. A prospective study of 2 major age-related macular degeneration susceptibility alleles and interactions with modifiable risk factors. *Arch Ophthalmol* 2007;125(1):55.

74. Stone EM. Genetic testing for inherited eye disease. *Arch Ophthalmol* 2007;125(2):205.

75. Grassi MA, Folk JC, Scheetz TE, et al. Complement factor H polymorphism p.Tyr402His and cuticular drusen. *Arch Ophthalmol* 2007; 125(January):93.

76. Anderson DH, Mullins RF, Hageman GS, et al. A role for local inflammation in the formation of drusen in the aging eye. *Am J Ophthalmol* 2002;134:411.

77. Seddon JE, Gensler G, Milton RC, et al. Association between C-reactive protein and age-related macular degeneration. *JAMA* 2004;291:704.

78. Vine AK, Stader J, Branham K, et al. Biomarkers of cardiovascular disease as risk factors for age-related macular degeneration. *Ophthalmology* 2005;112:2076.

79. Klein R, Klein BE, Knudtson MD, et al. Systemic markers of inflammation, endothelial dysfunction, and age-related maculopathy. *Am J Ophthalmol* 2005;140:35.

80. Rochtchina E, Wang JJ, Flood VM, et al. Elevated serum homocysteine, low serum vitamin B12, folate, and age-related macular degeneration: The Blue Mountains Eye Study. *Am J Ophthalmol* 2007;143 (2):344.

81. Klein R, Klein BE, Tomany SC, et al. Association of emphysema, gout, and inflammatory markers with long-term incidence of age-related maculopathy. *Arch Ophthalmol* 2003;121:674.

81b. Despriet DD, Klauver CC, Witteman JC, et al. Complement factor H polymorphism, complement activators and risk of age-related macular degeneration. *JAMA* 2006; 296(3):301–309.

82. Johnson LV, Anderson DH. Age-related macular degeneration and the extracellular matrix. *N Eng J Med* 2004;351:320.

83. Ferrara N, Houck K, Jakeman L, et al. Molecular and biological properties of the vascular endothelial growth factor family of proteins. *Endocr Rev* 1992;13:18.

84. Ferrara N. Vascular endothelial growth factor: Basic science and clinical progress. *Endocr Rev* 2004;25:581.

85. Grossniklaus HE, Ling JX, Wallace TM, et al. Macrophage and retinal pigment epithelium expression of angiogenic cytokines in choroidal neovascularization. *Mol Vis* 2002;8:119.

86. Spilsbury K, Garrett KL, Wei-Yong S, et al. Overexpression of vascular endothelial growth factor (VEGF) in retinal pigment epithelium leads to the development of choroidal neovascularization. *Am J Pathol* 2000;157:135.

87. Churchill AJ, Carter JG, Lovell HC, et al. VEGF polymorphisms are associated with neovascular age-related macular degeneration. *Hum Mol Genet* 2006;15(19):2955.

88. Age-Related Eye Disease Study Research Group. A randomized, placebo-controlled, clinical trial of high-dose supplementation with vitamins C and E, beta carotene, and zinc for age-related macular degeneration and vision loss: AREDS Report No. 8. *Arch Ophthalmol* 2001;119:1417–1436.

89. Submacular Surgery Trials Research Group. Responsiveness of the National Eye Institute Visual Function Questionnaire to changes in visual acuity: Findings in patients with subfoveal choroidal neovascularization. SST report no. 1. *Arch Ophthalmol* 2003;121:531–539.

90. Kuyk T, Elliott JL. Visual factors and mobility in persons with age-related macular degeneration. *J Rehabil Res Dev* 1999;36:303–312.

91. McClure ME, Hart PM, Jackson AJ, et al. Macular degeneration: Do conventional measurements of impaired visual function equate with visual disability? *Br J Ophthalmol* 2000;84:244–250.

92. Ergun E, Maar N, Radner W, et al. Scotoma size and reading speed in patients with subfoveal occult choroidal neovascularization in age-related macular degeneration. *Ophthalmology* 2003;110(1):65–69.

93. Sabates NR, Crane WG, Sabates FN, et al. Scanning laser ophthalmoscope macular perimetry in the evaluation of submacular surgery. *Retina* 1996;16(4):296–304.

94. Rohrschneider K, Gluck R, Becker M, et al. Scanning laser fundus perimetry before laser photocoagulation of well defined choroidal neovascularization. *Br J Ophthalmol* 1997;81:568–573.

95. Oshima Y, Harino S, Tano Y. Scanning laser ophthalmoscope microperimetric assessment in patients with successful laser treatment for juxtafoveal choroidal neovascularization. *Retina* 1998;18(2):109-117.

96. Alster Y, Bressler NM, Bressler SB, et al. Preferential Hyperacuity perimeter (Preview PHP) for detecting choroidal neovascularization study. *Ophthalmology* 2005;112:1758–1765.

97. Macular Photocoagulation Study Group. Argon laser photocoagulation for neovascular maculopathy. Three-year results from randomized clinical trials. *Arch Ophthalmol* 1986;104:694–701.

98. Macular Photocoagulation Study Group. Krypton laser photocoagulation for neovascular lesions of age-related macular degeneration. Results of a randomized clinical trial. *Arch Ophthalmol* 1990;108:816–824.

99. Macular Photocoagulation Study Group.: Laser photocoagulation of subfoveal neovascular lesions in age-related macular degeneration. Results of a randomized clinical trial. *Arch Ophthalmol* 1991;109: 1219–1230.

100. Zawinka C, Ergun E, Stur M. Prevalence of patients presenting with neovascular age-related macular degeneration in an urban population. *Retina* 2005;25:324–331.

101. Treatment of Age-Related Macular Degeneration with Photodynamic Therapy (TAP) and Verteporfin in Photodynamic (VIP) Study Groups. Photodynamic therapy of subfoveal choroidal neovascularization with verteporfin: Fluorescein angiographic guidelines for evaluation and treatment—TAP and VIP report no. 2. *Arch Ophthalmol* 2003; 121:1253–1268.

102. Macular Photocoagulation Study Group. Subfoveal neovascular lesions in age-related macular degeneration: Guidelines for evaluation and treatment in the Macular Photocoagulation Study. *Arch Ophthalmol* 1991;109:1242–1257.

103. Bressler SB, Pieramici DJ, Koester JM, et al. Natural history of minimally classic subfoveal choroidal neovascular lesions in the treatment of age-related macular degeneration with photodynamic therapy (TAP) investigation. Outcomes Potentially Relevant to Management—TAP Report No. 6. *Arch Ophthalmol* 2004;122:325–329.

104. Barbazetto I, Burdan A, Bressler NM, et al. Photodynamic therapy of subfoveal choroidal neovascularization with verteporfin: fluorescein

angiographic guidelines for evaluation and treatment—TAP and VIP report No. 2. *Arch Ophthalmol* 2003;121:1253–1268.

105. Treatment of Age-Related Macular Degeneration with Photodynamic Therapy (TAP) and Verteporfin in Photodynamic (VIP) Study Groups. Effect of lesion size, visual acuity, and lesion composition on visual acuity change with and without verteporfin therapy for choroidal neovascularization secondary to age-related macular degeneration: TAP and VIP report no. 1. *Am J Ophthalmol* 2003;136:407–418.

106. Fine SL, Berger JW, Maguire MG. Age-related macular degeneration. *N Engl J Med* 2000;342:483–492.

107. Costa RA, Farah ME, Cardillo JA. Immediate indocyanine green angiography and optical coherence tomography evaluation after photodynamic therapy for subfoveal choroidal neovascularization. *Retina* 2003;23(2):159–165.

108. Fernandes LH, Freund KB, Yanuzzi LA, et al. The nature of focal areas of hyperfluorescence or hot spots imaged with indocyanine green angiography. *Retina* 2002;22:557–568.

109. Macular Photocoagulation Study Group. Argon laser photocoagulation for neovascular maculopathy: three-year results from randomized clinical trials. *Arch Ophthalmol* 1986;104:694.

110. Macular Photocoagulation Study Group. Krypton laser photocoagulation for neovascular lesions of age-related macular degeneration: results of a randomized clinical trial. *Arch Ophthalmol* 1990;108:816–824.

111. Macular Photocoagulation Study Group. Argon laser photocoagulation for neovascular maculopathy: five-year results from randomized clinical trials. *Arch Ophthalmol* 1991;109:1109.

112. Macular Photocoagulation Study Group. Laser photocoagulation Study Group. Laser photocoagulation of subfoveal neovascular lesions in age-related macular degeneration: results of randomized clinical trial. *Arch Ophthalmol* 1991;109:1220.

113. Macular Photocoagulation Study Group. Subfoveal neovascular lesions in age-related macular degeneration: guidelines for evaluation and treatment in the Macular Photocoagulation Study. *Arch Ophthalmol* 1991;109:1242.

114. Macular Photocoagulation Study Group. Laser photocoagulation of subfoveal neovascular lesions of age-related macular degeneration:

updated findings from two clinical trials. *Arch Ophthalmol* 1993;111: 1200.

115. Macular Photocoagulation Study Group. Laser photocoagulation for juxtafoveal choroidal neovascularization: five-year results from randomized clinical trials. *Arch Ophthalmol* 1994;112:500.

116. Macular Photocoagulation Study Group. Visual outcome after laser photocoagulation for subfoveal choroidal neovascularization secondary to age-related macular degeneration: the influence of initial lesion size and initial visual acuity. *Arch Ophthalmol* 1994;112:480.

117. Macular Photocoagulation Study Group. Occult choroidal neovascularization: influence on visual outcome in patients with age-related macular degeneration. *Arch Ophthalmol* 1996;114:400.

118. Fruend KB, Yannuzzi L, Sorenson JA. Age-related macular degeneration and choroidal neovascularization. *Am J Ophthalmol* 1993;115 (6):786.

119. Margherio RR, Margherio AR, DeSantis ME. Laser treatment with verteporfin therapy and its potential impact on retinal practices. *RETINA* 2000;20(4):325.

120. Treatment of Age-Related Macular Degeneration with Photodynamic Therapy (TAP) Study Group. Photodynamic therapy of subfoveal choroidal neovascularization in age-related macular degeneration with verteporfin: One-year results of 2 randomized clinical trials-TAP Report No. 1. *Arch Ophthalmol* 1999; 117:1329.

121. Schmidt-Erfurth U, Schlotzer-Schrehard U, Cursiefen C, et al. Influence of photodynamic therapy on expression of vascular endothelial growth factor (VEGF), VEGF receptor 3, and pigment epithelium-derived factor. *Invest Ophthalmol Vis Sci* 2003;44:4473.

122. Costa RA, Farah ME, Cardillo JA, et al. Immediate indocyanine green angiography and optical coherence tomography evaluation after photodynamic therapy for subfoveal choroidal neovascularization. *RETINA* 2003 23:159.

123. Bressler NM. Treatment of age-Related Macular Degeneration With Photodynamic Therapy (TAP) Study Group. Photodynamic therapy of subfoveal choroidal neovascularization in age-related macular degeneration with verteporfin: Two-year results of 2 randomized clinical trials-TAP Report 2. *Arch Ophthalmol* 2001;119:198.

124. Bressler NM. Photodynamic therapy of subfoveal choroidal neovascularization in age-related macular degeneration with verteporfin: Two-year results of 2 randomized clinical trials-TAP Report No. 2. *Arch Ophthalmol* 2001;119:198.

125. Bressler NM, Arnold JJ, Benchaboune M, et al. Verteporfin therapy of subfoveal choroidal neovascularization in patients with age-related macular degeneration: additional information regarding baseline lesion composition's impact on vision outcomes-TAP Report No. 3. *Arch Ophthalmol* 2002;120:1443.

126. Blumenkranz MS, Bressler NM, Bressler SB, et al. Verteporfin therapy for subfoveal choroidal neovascularization in age-related macular degeneration: three-year results of an open-label extension of 2 randomized clinical trials-TAP Report No. 5. *Arch Ophthalmol* 2002;120:1307.

127. Verteporfin In Photodynamic Therapy Study Group. Verteporfin therapy of subfoveal choroidal neovascularization in age-related macular degeneration: Two-year results of a randomized clinical trial including lesions with occult with no classic choroidalneovascularization-verteporfin in photodynamic therapy Report No. 2. *Am J Ophthalmol* 2001;131:541.

128. Blinder KJ, Bradley S, Bressler NM, et al. Effect of lesion size, visual acuity, and lesion composition on visual acuity change with and without verteporfin therapy for choroidal neovascularization secondary to age-related macular degeneration: TAP and VIP Report No.1. *Am J Ophthalmol* 2003;136:407.

129. Azab M, Benchaboune M, Blinder KJ, et al. Verteporfin therapy of subfoveal choroidal neovascularization in age-related macular degeneration: meta-analysis of 2-year safety results in three randomized clinical trials: Treatment of Age-Related Macular Degeneration With Photodynamic Therapy and Verteporfin in Photodynamic Therapy Study Report No. 4. *RETINA* 2004;24:1.

130. Azab M, Boyer DS, Bressler NM, et al. Verteporfin therapy of subfoveal minimally classic choroidal neovascularization in age-related macular degeneration: 2-year results of a randomized clinical trial. *Arch Ophthalmol* 2005;123:448.

131. Boyer DS, Antoszyk AN, Awh CC, et al. Subgroup analysis of the MARINA Study of ranibizumab in neovascular age-related macular degeneration. *Ophthalmology* 2007;114:246.

132. Rosenfeld P. The Visudyne in Minimally Classic CNV (VIM) Study Group. *Invest Ophthalmol Vis Sci* 2004. 45(E-Abstract):2273.

133. Arnold JJ, Blinder KJ, Bressler NM, et al. Acute severe visual acuity decrease after photodynamic therapy with vereporfin: case reports from randomized clinical trials - TAP and VIP Report No. 3. *Am J Ophthalmol* 2004;137:683.

134. Conti SM, Kertes PJ. Surgical management of age-related macular degeneration. *Can J Ophthalmol* 2005;40(3):341.

135. Submacular Surgery Trials (SST) Research Group. Surgery for subfoveal choroidal neovascularization in age-related macular degeneration: Ophthalmic findings. SST Report No. 11. *Ophthalmology* 2004;111:1967.

136. Submacular Surgery Trials (SST) Research Group. Surgery for hemorrhagic choroidal neovascular lesions of age-related macular degeneration: Ophthalmic findings. SST Report No. 13. *Ophthalmology* 2004. 111:1993.

137. Haupert CL, McCuen BW, II Jaffe GJ, et al. Pars plana vitrectomy, subretinal injection of tissue plasminogen activator, and fluid-gas exchange for displacement of thick submacular hemorrhage in age-related macular degeneration. *Am J Ophthalmol* 2001; 131(2):208.

138. Olivier S, Chow DR, Packo KH, et al. Subretinal recombinant tissue plasminogen activator injection and pneumatic displacement of thick submacular hemorrhage in age-related macular degeneration. *Ophthalmology* 2004;111(6):1201.

139. Au Eong KG, Pieramici DJ, Fujii GY, et al. Macular translocation: unifying concepts, terminology, and classification. *Am J Ophthalmol* 2001;131(2):244.

140. Eckardt C, Eckardt U, Conrad HG. Macular rotation with and without counter-rotation of the globe in patients with age-related macular degeneration. *Graefes Arch Clin Exp Ophthalmol* 1999;237(4):313.

141. Fujii GY, Au Eong KG, Humayun MS, et al. Limited macular translocation: current concepts. *Ophthalmol Clin North Am* 2002;15(4):425.

142. Kamei M, Tano Y, Yasuhara T, et al. Macular translocation with chorioscleral outfolding: 2-year results. *Am J Ophthalmol* 2004;138(4): 574.

143. Cahill MT, Banks AD, Stinnett SS, et al. Vision-related quality of life in patients with bilateral severe age-related macular degeneration. *Ophthalmology* 2005;112:152.

144. Cahill MT, Stinnett SS, Banks AD, et al. Quality of life after macular translocation with 360 degrees peripheral retinectomy for age-related macular degeneration. *Ophthalmology* 2005;112(1):144.

145. Toth CA, Lapolice DJ, Banks AD, et al. Improvement in near visual function after macular translocation surgery with 360 degree peripheral retinectomy. *Graefes Arch Clin Exp Ophthalmol* 2004;242(7):541.

146. Abdel-Meguid A, Lappas A, Hartmann K, et al. One year follow up of macular translocation with 360 degree retinopathy in patients with age related macular degeneration. *Br J Ophthalmol* 2003;87(5):615.

147. Del Priore LV, Tezel TH, Kaplan HJ. Maculoplasty for age-related macular degeneration: reengineering Bruch's membrane and the human macula. *Prog Retin Eye Res* 2006;25(6):539.

148. Staurenghi G, Orzalesi N, La Capria A, Aschero M. Laser treatment of feeder vessels in subfoveal choroidal neovascular membranes: A revisitation using dynamic indocyanine green angiography. *Ophthalmology* 1998;105(12):2297.

149. Spaide RF, Sorenson J, Maranan L. Combined photodynamic therapy with verteporfin and intravitreal triamcinolone acetonide for choroidal neovascularization. *Ophthalmology* 2003;110:1517.

150. Spaide RF, Sorenson J, Maranan L. Photodynamic therapy with verteporfin combined with intravitreal injection of traimcinolone acetonide for choroidal neovascularization. *Ophthalmology* 2005;112:301.

151. Augustin AJ, Puls S, Offerman I. Triple therapy for choroidal neovascularization due to age-related macular degeneration. Verteporfin PDT, Bevacizumab, and Dexamethasone. *Retina* 2007;26:133.

152. Costa RA, Jorge R, Calucci D, et al. Intravitreal bevacizumab (Avastin) in combination with verteporfin photodynamic therapy for choroidal neovascularization associated with age-related macular degeneration (IBeVe Study). *Graefes Arch Clin Exp Ophthalmol* 2007. epub ahead of print.

153. Dhalla MS, Shah GK, Blinder KJ, et al. Combined photodynamic therapy with verteporfin and intravitreal bevacizumab for choroidal neovascularization in age-related macular degeneration. *Retina* 2006;26:988.

154. Gragoudas ES, Adamis AP, Cunningham ET, et al. VEGF Inhibition Study in Ocular Neovascularization Clinical Trial Group. Pegaptanib for neovascular age-related macular degeneration. *N Engl J Med* 2004;351:2805–2816.

155. Zhou B, Wang B. Pegaptanib for the treatment of age-related macular degeneration. *Exp Eye Res* 2006;83:615–619.

156. Gonzales CR. The VEGF Inhibition Study in Ocular Neovascularization (VISION) Clinical Trial Group. Enhanced efficacy associated with early treatment of neovascular age-related macular degeneration with pegaptanib sodium: an exploratory analysis. *Retina* 2005;25:815–827.

157. Ferrara N, Hillan KJ, Gerber HP, et al. Discovery and development of bevacizumab, an anti-VEGF antibody for treating cancer. *Nat Rev Drug Discov* 2004;3:391–400.

158. Chen Y, Wiesmann C, Fuh G, et al. Selection and analysis of an optimized anti-VEGF antibody: Crystal structure of an affinity-matured Fab in complex with antigen. *J Mol Biol* 1999;293:865–881.

159. Presta LG, Chen H, O'Connor SJ, et al. Humanization of an anti-vascular endothelial growth factor monoclonal antibody for the therapy of solid tumors and other disorders. *Cancer Res* 1997;57:4593–4599.

160. Krzystolik MG, Afshari MA, Adamis AP, et al. Prevention of experimental choroidal neovascularization with intravitreal anti-vascular endothelial growth factor antibody fragment. *Arch Ophthalmol* 2002;120:338–346.

161. Gaudreault J, Fei D, Rusit J, et al. Preclinical pharmacokinetics of ranibizumab (rhuFab V2) after a single intravitreal administration. *Invest Ophthalmol Vis Sci* 2005;46:726–733.

162. Rosenfeld PJ, Heier JS, Hantsbarger G, et al. Tolerability and efficacy of multiple escalating doses of ranibizumab for neovascular age-related macular degeneration. *Ophthalmology* 2006;113:632e1.

163. Heier JS, Antoszyk AN, Pavan PR, et al. Ranibizumab for treatment of neovascular age-related macular degeneration: A phase I/II multicenter, controlled, multidose study. *Ophthalmology* 2006;113:642.e1–e4.

164. Rosenfeld PJ, Schwartz SD, Blumenkranz MS, et al. Maximum tolerated dose of a humanized anti-vascular endothelial growth factor antibody fragment for treating neovascular age-related macular degeneration. *Ophthalmology* 2005;112:1048–1053.

165. Rosenfeld PJ, Brown DM, Heier JS, et al for The Marina Study Group. Ranibizumab for neovascular age-related macular degeneration. *N Engl J Med* 2006;355:1419–1431.

166. Brown DM, Kaiser PK, Michels M, et al for The Anchor Study Group. Ranibizumab versus verteporfin for neovascular age-related macular degeneration. *N Engl J Med* 2006;355:1432–1444.

167. Data on file, Genentech, Inc.

168. Brown DM, Shapior H, Schneider S, et al. Subgroup analysis of first-year results of ANCHOR: A phase III, double-masked, randomized, comparison of ranibizumab and verteporfin photodynamic therapy for predominantly classic choroidal neovascularization related to age-related macular degeneration. Presented at: Annual Meeting of the Association for Research in Vision and Ophthalmology; April 30–May 4, 2006; Fort Lauderdale, Florida.

169. Heier JS, Boyer DS, Ciulla TA, et al. Ranibizumab combined with verteporfin photodynamic therapy in neovascular age-related macular degeneration: year 1 results of the FOCUS Study. *Arch Ophthalmol* 2006;124(11):1532–1542.

170. Michels S, Rosenfeld PJ, Puliafito CA, et al. Systemic bevacizumab (Avastin) therapy for neovascular age-related macular degeneration twelve-week results of an uncontrolled open-label clinical study. *Ophthalmology* 2005;112:1035–1047.

171. Rosenfeld PJ, Moshfeghi AA, Puliafito CA. Optical coherence tomography findings after an intravitreal injection of bevacizumab (Avastin®) for neovascular age-related macular degeneration. *Ophthalmic Surg Lasers Imaging* 2005;36:331–335.

172. Avery RL, Pieramici DJ, Rabena MD, et al. Intravitreal bevacizumab for neovascular age-related macular degeneration. *Ophthalmology* 2006;113:363–372.e.5

173. Spaide RF, Laud K, Fine HF, et al. Intravitreal bevacizumab treatment of choroidal neovascularization secondary to age-related macular degeneration. *Retina* 2006;26:383–390.

174. Bashshur ZF, Bazarbachi A, Schakal A, et al. Intravitreal bevacizumab for the management of choroidal neovascularization in age-related macular degeneration. *Am J Ophthalmol* 2006;142:1–9.

175. Maturi RK, Bleau LA, Wildon DL. Electrophysiologic findings after intravitreal bevacizumab treatment. *Retina* 2006;26:270–274.

176. Fung AE, Rosenfeld PJ, Reichel EZ. Intravitreal Avastin safety survey: results from the world wide web. *Invest Ophthalmol Vis Sci* 2006;47ARVO E-abstract 5251.

177. Mangione CM, Lee PP, Gutierrez PR, et al. National Eye Institute Visual Function Questionnaire Field Test Investigators. Development of the 25-item National Eye Institute Visual Function Questionnaire. *Arch Ophthalmol* 2001;119:1050–1058.

178. Lindblad AS, Clemons TE. Responsiveness of the National Eye Institute Visual Function Questionnaire to progression to advanced age-related macular degeneration, vision loss, and lens opacity. AREDS Report no. 14. *Arch Ophthalmol* 2005;123:1207–1214.

179. Miskala PH, Bressler NM, Meinert CL. Relative contributions of reduced vision and general health to NEI-VFQ scores in patients with neovascular age-related macular degeneration. *Arch Ophthalmol* 2004;122:758–766.

180. Holash J, Davis S, Papadopoulos N, et al. VEGF-Trap: A VEGF blocker with potent antitumor effects. *PNAS* 2002;99(12): 11393–11398.

181. Nguyen D, Shah SM, Browning D, et al. Results of a phase I, dose-escalation, safety, tolerability, and bioactivity study of intravitreous VEGF Trap in patients with neovascular age-related macular degeneration. Presented at the Annual Meeting of the Association for Research in Vision and Ophthalmology (ARVO); April 30–May 4, 2006; Fort Lauderdale, Florida.

182. Fire A, Xu S, Montgomery MK, et al. Potent and specific genetic interference by double-stranded RNA in Caenorhabditis elegans. *Nature* 1998;391:6669:806–811.

183. Shen C, Andreas KB, Liu X, et al. Gene silencing by adenovirus siRNA. *Federation of European Biochemical Societies Letters* 2003;539:111–114.

184. Devroe E, Silver PA. Retrovirus-delivered siRNA. *BMC Biotechnology* 2002;2:15.

185. Data, Acuity Pharmaceuticals. Available at: www.acuitypharma.com/press/release15.pdf.

186. McCain J. Renewing the assault on mRNA. *Biotechnol Healthcare* 2004;1:44–53.

187. SiRNA Therapeutics. SiRNA Therapeutics announces results from interim analysis of phase I single-dose trial with SiRNA-027 in patients with age-related macular degeneration (press release). www.biospace.com/news_story.aspx?storyID=19935020&full=1.

188. Genaera Corporation. Clinical results presented for Evizon (squalamine lactate) for treatment of age-related macular degeneration (press release). Available at www.pslgroup.com/dg/24f2e2.htm.

189. Schmidt-Erfurth U, Schlotzer-Schrehard U, Cursiefen C, et al. Influence of photodynamic therapy on expression of vascular endothelial growth factor (VEGF), VEGF receptor 3, and pigment epithelium-derived factor. *Invest Ophthalmol Vis Sci* 2003;44:4473–4480.

190. Stellmach V, Crawford SE, Zhou W, et al. Prevention of ischemia-induced retinopathy by the natural ocular antiangiogenic agent pigment epithelium-derived factor. *Proc Natl Acad Sci USA* 2001;98:2593–2597.

191. Mori K, Gehlbach P, Yamamoto S, et al. AAV-mediated gene transfer of pigment epithelium-derived factor inhibits choroidal neovascularization. *Invest Ophthalmol Vis Sci* 2002;43:1994–2000.

192. GenVec, Inc. AdPEDF for Macular Degeneration. Available at www.genvec.com/go.cfm?do=Page.View&pid=30.

193. Campochiaro PA, Nguyen QD, Shah SM, et al. Adenoviral vector-delivered pigment epithelium-derived factor for neovascular age-related macular degeneration: Results of a phase I clinical trial. *Hum Gene Ther* 2006;17:167–176.

194. Kinose F, Roscilli G, Lamartina S,. et al. Inhibition of retinal and choroidal neovascularization by a novel KDR kinase inhibitor. *Molecular Vision.* 2005;11:366–373.

195. Maier P, Unsoeld A, Junker B, et al. Intravitreal injection of specific receptor tyrosine kinase inhibitor PTK787/ZK222 584 improves ischemia-induced retinopathy in mice. *Arch Clin Exp Ophthalmol* 2005;243:593–600.

196. OxiGENE, Inc. Combretastatin. New research highlights a novel mechanism of action for OXiGENE's lead vascular disrupting agent, CA4P. Available at www.oxigene.com/press/pressreleases.asp.

197. Vincent l, Kermani P, Young LM, et al. Combretastatin A4 phosphate induces rapid regression of tumor neovessels and growth through interference with vascular endothelial-cadherin signaling. *J Clin Invest* 2005;115:2992–3006.

198. Friberg TR, PTAMD Study Group. The Prophylactic Treatment of AMD Multi-Centered Trial (PTAMD): results from the bilateral study arm. *Invest Ophthalmol Vis* Sci 2006;47:ARVO E-abstract 3538.

199. Friberg TR, Musch DC, Lim Jl, et al. Prophylactic treatment of age-related macular degeneration report number 1: 810 nanometer laser to eyes with drusen. Unilaterally eligible patients. *Ophthalmology* 2006;113:612–622.

200. Hudson HL, Lane SS, Heier JS, et al for the IMT-002 Study Group. Implantable miniature telescope for the treatment of visual acuity loss resulting from end-stage age-related macular degeneration. *Ophthalmology* 2006;113:1987–2001.

201. Finger PT, Berson A, Sherr D, et al. Radiation therapy for subretinal neovascularization. *Ophthalmology* 1996 Jun; 103(6):878–889.

202. Finger PT, Berson A, Ng T, et al. Ophthalmic plaque radiotherapy for age-related macular degeneration associated with subretinal neovascularization. *Am J Ophthalmol* 1999;127(2):170–177.

203. Yonemoto LT, Slater JD, Friedrichsen EJ, et al Phase I/II study of proton beam irradiation for the treatment of subfoveal choroidal neovascularization in age-related macular degeneration: treatment techniques and preliminary results. *Int J Radiat Oncol Biol Phys* 1996;36(4): 867–871.

204. Anders N, Stahl H, Dorn A, et al. Radiotherapy of exudative senile macular degeneration. A prospective controlled study. *Ophthalmologe* 1998; 95(11): 760–764.

205. Char DH, Irvine AI, Posner MD, et al. Randomized trial of radiation for age-related macular degeneration. *Am J Ophthalmol* 1999; 127(5): 574–578.

206. Krott R, Staar S, Muller RP, et al. External beam radiation in patients suffering from exudative age-related macular degeneration. A matched-pairs study and 1-year clinical follow-up. *Graefes Arch Clin Exp Ophthalmol* 1998; 236(12): 916–921.

207. Mauget-Faysse M, Chiquet C, Milea D, et al. Long term results of radiotherapy for subfoveal choroidal neovascularisation in age related macular degeneration. *Br J Ophthalmol* 1999; 83(8): 923–928.

208. Subasi M, Akmansu M, Or M. Treatment of age-related subfoveal neovascular membranes by teletherapy: results of a non-randomized study. *Radiat Med* 1999 Mar-Apr; 17(2): 169–173.

209. Tholen AM, Meister A, Bernasconi PP, et al. Radiotherapy for choroidal neovascularization in age-related macular degeneration. A pilot study using low- versus high-dose photon bean radiation. *Ophthalmologe* 1998; 95(10): 691–698.

210. Spaide R: External beam radiation therapy for choroidal neovascularization. Paper presented at: International Symposium on Radiation Therapy for Macular Degeneration; 1997; New York, NY.

211. Spaide RF, Guyer DR, McCormick B, et al. External beam radiation therapy for choroidal neovascularization. *Ophthalmology* 1998; 105(1): 24–30.

212. Roesen B, Scheider A, Kiraly A, et al. Choroid neovascularization in senile macular degeneration. 1 year follow-up after radiotherapy. *Ophthalmologe* 1998; 95(7): 461–465.

213. Weinberger AW, Wolf S, Kube T, et al. Radiation therapy of occult choroidal neovascularisation (CNV) in age-related macular degeneration (AMD). *Klin Monatsbl Augenheilkd* 1999; 214(2): 96–99.

214. RAD Study Group. A prospective, randomized, double-masked trial on radiation therapy for neovascular age-related macular degeneration (RAD Study). Radiation Therapy for Age-related Macular Degeneration. *Ophthalmology* 1999; 106(12): 2239–2247.

215. Marcus DM, Sheils W, Johnson MH, et al. External beam irradiation of subfoveal choroidal neovascularization complicating age-related macular degeneration: one-year results of a prospective, double-masked, randomized clinical trial. *Arch Ophthalmol* 2001; 119(2): 171–180.

216. Bergink GJ, Hoyng CB, van der Maazen RW, et al. A randomized controlled clinical trial on the efficacy of radiation therapy in the control of subfoveal choroidal neovascularization in age-related macular degeneration: radiation versus observation. *Graefes Arch Clin Exp Ophthalmol* 1998; 236(5): 321–325.

217. Char DH, Irvine AI, Posner MD, et al. Randomized trial of radiation for age-related macular degeneration. *Am J Ophthalmol* 1999; 127(5): 574–578.

218. Marcus D, Peskin E, Alexander J, et al. The age-related macular degeneration radiotherapy trial (AMDRT): 1-year results [E-abstract]. *Invest Ophthalmol Vis Sci* 2003; 44:3158.

219. Ciulla TA, Harris A, Kagemann L, et al. Transpupillary thermotherapy for subfoveal occult choroidal neovascularization: effect on ocular perfusion. *Invest Ophthalmol Vis Sci* 2001; 42(13):3337–3340.

220. Kroll P, Meyer CH. Which treatment is best for which AMD patient? *Br J Ophthalmol* 2006;90:128–130.

221. Miura S, Nishiwaki H, Ieki Y, et al. Chorioretinal temperature monitoring during Transpupillary thermotherapy for choroidal neovascularization. *Br J Ophthalmol* 2005;89(11):1545.

222. Reichel E, Berrocal AM, Ip M, et al. Transpupillary thermotherapy of occult subfoveal choroidal neovascularization in patients with age-related macular degeneration. *Ophthalmology* 1999; 106(10):1908–1914.

223. Thach AB, Sipperley JO, Dugel PU, et al. Large-spot size transpupillary thermotherapy for the treatment of occult choroidal neovascularization associated with age-related macular degeneration. *Arch Ophthalmol* 2003; 121(6):817–820.

224. VIP Study Group. Verteporfin therapy of subfoveal choroidal neovascularization in age-related macular degeneration: Two-year results of a randomized clinical trial including lesions with occult with no classic choroidal neovascularization. *Am J Ophthalmol* 2001; 131(5): 541–560.

225. Nader N. Clinical trials show promise of intravitreal steroids, other therapies for retinal diseases. *Ocular Surg News* 2004; 22(3):28–30.

226. Schultz J. Significant clinical benefit of TTT seen in subset of patients in CNV trial. *Ocular Surgery News* 2005; 23(8): 56–57.

227. Stolba U, Krebs I, Lamar PD, et al. Long term results after Transpupillary thermotherapy in eyes with occult choroidal neovascularization associated with age-related macular degeneration: A prospective trial. *Br J Ophthalmol* 2006;90:158–161.

228. Crum R, Szabo S, Folkman J. A new class of steroids inhibits angiogenesis in the presence of heparin or a heparin fragment. *Science* 1985; 230(4732): 1375–1378.

229. Clark AF, Mellon J, Li XY, et al. Inhibition of intraocular tumor growth by topical application of the angiostatic steroid anecortave acetate. *Invest Ophthalmol Vis Sci* 1999; 40(9): 2158–2162.

230. Penn JS, Rajaratnam VS, Collier RJ, et al. The effect of an angiostatic steroid on neovascularization in a rat model of retinopathy of prematurity. *Invest Ophthalmol Vis Sci* 2001; 42(1): 283–290.

231. Alcon Laboratories, Inc. Alcon receives approvable letter from FDA for RETAANE suspension [Alcon Laboratories, Inc Web site]. May 24, 2005. Available at: http://invest.alconinc.com/phoenix.zhtml?c=130946&p=irol-newsArticle&ID=713392&highlight.

232. Slakter JS, Bochow TW, D'Amico DJ, et al. Anecortave acetate (15 milligrams) versus photodynamic therapy for treatment of subfoveal neovascularization in age-related macular degeneration. *Ophthalmology* 2006;113:3–13.

233. Chew EY, Clemons T. Vitamin E and the age-related eye disease study supplementation for age-related macular degeneration. *Arch Ophthalmol* 2005;123:395–396.

234. van Leeuwen R, Boekhoorn S, Vingerling JR, et al. Dietary intake of antioxidants and risk of age-related macular degeneration. *JAMA* 2005;294:3101–3107.

235. Clemons TE, Milton RC, Klein R, et al. Risk factors for the incidence of advanced age-related macular degeneration in the age-related eye disease study (AREDS). AREDS Report no. 19. *Ophthalmology* 2005;112:533–539.

236. Tomany SC, Wang JJ, van Leewen R, et al. Risk factors for incident age-related macular degeneration: Pooled findings from 3 continents. *Ophthalmology* 2004;111:1280–1287.

237. Seddon JM, Cote J, Page WF. The US Twin Study of Age-Related Macular Degeneration: Relative roles of genetic and environmental influences. *Arch Ophthalmol* 2005;123:321–327.

238. Ambati J, Ambati BK, Yoo SH, et al. Age-related macular degeneration: etiology, pathogenesis, and therapeutic strategies. *Surv Ophthalmol* 2003;48:257–293.

239. Seddon JM, Cote J, Davis N, et al. Progression of age-related macular degeneration: association with body mass index, waist circumference, and waist-hip ratio. *Arch Ophthalmol* 2003;121:785–792.

240. Seddon JM, Cote J, Rosner B. Progression of age-related macular degeneration: association with dietary fat, transunsaturated fat, nuts, and fish intake. *Arch Ophthalmol* 2003;121:1728–1737.

241. Cho E, Hung S, Willett WC, et al. Prospective study of dietary fat and the risk of age-related macular degeneration. *Am J Clin Nutr* 2001;73: 209–218.

242. Rosenthal J, San Giovanni JP, Agron E, et al. A dietary antioxidant index and risk for advanced age-related macular degeneration in the Age-Related Eye Disease Study. Paper presented at the Annual Meeting of the Association for Research in Vision and Ophthalmology; April 30–May 4, 2006. Ft. Lauderdale, Florida.

243. Moeller SM, Parekh N, Tinker L, et al. Associations between intermediate age-related macular degeneration and lutein and zeaxanthin in the Carotenoids in Age-Related Eye Disease Study (CAREDS). *Arch Opthalmol* 2006;124:1151–1162.

244. Knudtson MD, Klein R, Klein BE. Physical activity and the 15-year cumulative incidence of age-related macular degeneration. The Beaver Dam Eye Study. *Br J Ophthalmol* 2006;90(12)1461–1463.

245. Altman DG. Confidence intervals for the number needed to treat. *Br J Ophthalmol* 1998;317:1309.

246. Rovner BW, Ganguli M. Depression and disability associated with impaired vision: the MoVies project. *J Am Geriatr So* 1998;46:617.

247. Dong LM, Childs AL, Mangione CM, et al. Health and vision-related quality of life among patients with choroidal neovascularization secondary to age-related macular degeneration at enrollment in randomized trials of submacular surgery. SST Report No. 4. *Am J Ophthalmol* 2004;138:91.

248. Evans 2007.

249. Park W. Vision rehabilitation for age-related macular degeneration. *Int Ophthalmol Clin* 1999;39:143.

250. Peli E, Goldstein RB, Young GM, et al. Image enhancement for the visually impaired. Simulations and experimental results. *Invest Ophthalmol Vis Sci* 1991;32:2337.

251. Slakter JS, Stur M. Quality of life in patients with age-related macular degeneration: impact on the condition and benefits of treatment. *Surv Opthalmol* 2005;50:263.

252. Mangione CM, Gutierrez PF, Lowe G, et al. Influence of age-related maculopathy on visual functioning and health-related quality of life. *Am J Ophthalmol* 1999;128:45.

253. Miskala PH, Hawkins BS, Mangione CM, et al. Responsiveness of the National Eye Institute Visual Function Questionnaire to changes in visual acuity: Findings in patients with subfoveal neovascularization - SST Report No. 1. *Arch Ophthalmol* 2003;121:531.

254. The Submacular Surgery Trials Research Group. Responsiveness of the National Eye Institute Visual Function Questionnaire to changes in visual acuity: Findings in patients with subfoveal choroidal neovascularization—SST Report No. 1. *Arch Ophthalmol* 2003;121(4):531.

255. Stevenson MR, Hart PM, Montgomery AM, et al. Reduced vision in older adults with age-related macular degeneration interferes with ability to care for self and impairs role as carer. *Ophthalmology* 2004; 88:1125.

256. Clemons TE, Rankin MW, McBee WL, et al. Cognitive impairment in the age-related eye disease study: AREDS report No. 16. *Arch Ophthalmol* 2006;124(4):537.

257. Pham TQ, Kifley A, Wang JJ. Relation of age-related macular degeneration and cognitive impairment in an older population. *Gerontology* 2006;52(6):353.

258. Brown GC, Brown NM, Sharma S. Difference between ophthalmologists' and patients' perceptions of quality of life associated with age-related macular degeneration. *Can J Ophthalmol* 2000;35:127–133.

259. Brown GC, Brown MM, Sharma S, et al. The burden of age-related macular degeneration: a value-based medicine analysis. *Trans Am Ophthalmol Soc* 2005;103:173.

260. Brown MM, Brown GC, Sharma S, et al. The burden of age-related macular degeneration: a value-based analysis. *Curr Opin Ophthalmol* 2006;17(3):257.

261. Brown GC, Brown MM, Campanella J, et al. The cost-utility of photodynamic therapy in eyes with neovascular macular degeneration—a value-based reappraisal with 5-year data. *Am J Ophthalmol* 2005;140(4):679.

262. Hopley C, Salkeld G, Mitchell P. Cost utility of photodynamic therapy for predominantly classic neovascular age related macular degeneration. *Br J Ophthalmol* 2004;88(8):982.

263. Bansback N, Davis S, Brazier J. Using contrast sensitivity to estimate the cost-effectiveness of verteporfin in patients with predominantly classic age-related macular degeneration. *Eye* 2006.

264. Smith DH, Fenn P, Drummond M. Cost effectiveness of photodynamic therapy with verteporfin for age related macular degeneration: The UK case. *Br J Ophthalmol* 2004;88(9):1107.

265. Sharma S, Oliver-Fernandez A. Age-related macular degeneration and quality of life: How to interpret a research paper in health-related quality of life. *Curr Opin Ophthalmol* 2004;15:227.

266. Sharma S, Hollands H, Brown GC, et al. Improvement in quality of life from photodynamic therapy: A Canadian perspective. *Can J Ophthalmol* 2001;36:332.

267. Armbrecht AM, Aspinall PA, Dhillon BA. A prospective study of visual function and quality of life following PDT in patients with wet age related macular degeneration. *Ophthalmology* 2004;88:1270.

268. Krummenauer F, Braun M, Dick HB. Clinical outcome and subjective quality of life after photodynamic therapy in patients with age-related macular degeneration. *Ophthalmology* 2005;15:74.

269. Chang TS. The importance of vision-related quality of life in patients treated for neovascular AMD. *Retina Today* 2007;2(1):17.

270. Bass EB, Marsh MJ, Mangione CM, et al. Patients' perceptions of the value of current vision: assessment of preference values among patients with subfoveal choroidal neovascularization- The Submacular Surgery Trials Vision Perception Value Scale. Submacular Surgery Trials Research Group (SST). *Arch Ophthalmol* 2004;122:1856.

271. Brown MM, Brown GC, Stein JD, et al. Age-related macular degeneration: Economic burden and value-based medicine analysis. *Can J Ophthalmol* 2005;40(3):277.

272. Javitt JC, Zhou Z, Wilke RJ. Association between vision loss and higher medical care costs in Medicare beneficiaries. Costs are greater for those with progressive vision loss. *Ophthalmology* 2007;114:238.

Index